DANCE FEVER

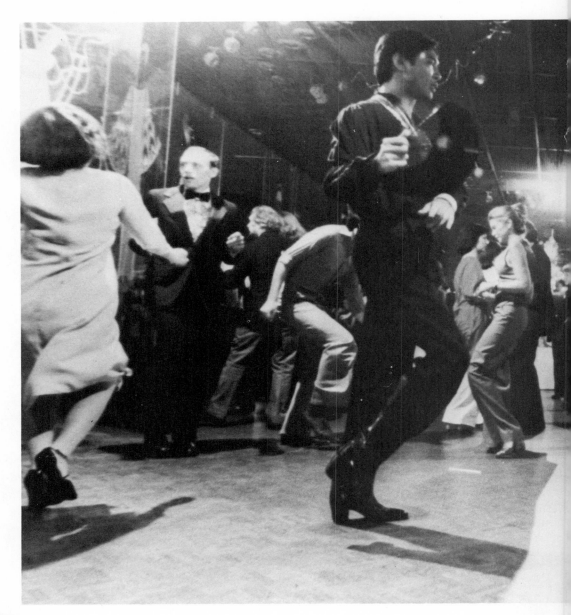

DANCE

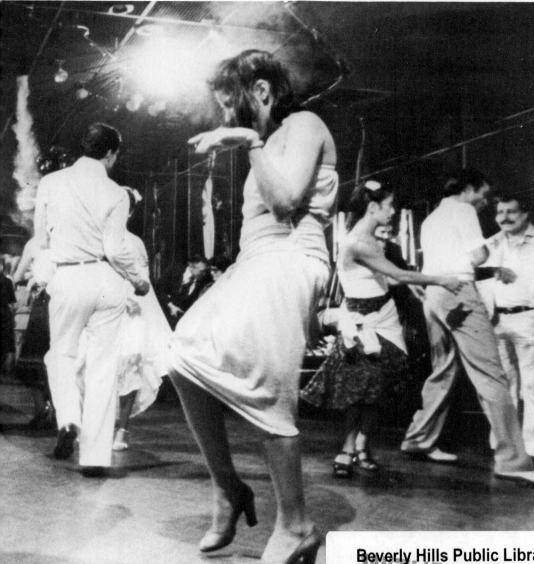

FEVER

by Don McDonagh

RANDOM HOUSE, INC. PUBLISHERS NEW YORK

For Jenny who likes dancing.

My thanks to Genevieve Oswald and the exceptionally
helpful staff of the Dance Collection, Performing
Arts Research Center, New York Public Library
at Lincoln Center, Astor, Lenox and Tilden Foundations,
for their assistance in locating films, publications
and newspaper clippings.

Produced and prepared by Quarto Marketing Ltd., New York
Editor: Anne Ziff
Associate Editor: Nancy McNally
Production Manager: Tammy O'Bradovich
Designed by Ruth Kolbert
Photo Research: Tricia Grantz

Original design concept by Ed Schneider

Library of Congress Cataloging in Publication Data

McDonagh, Don.
Dance fever.

Includes index.
1. Dancing—United States—History.   I.   Title.
GV1623.M27   793.3'1973   78-21812
ISBN 0-394-50410-0
ISBN 0-394-73667-0 pbk.

CONTENTS

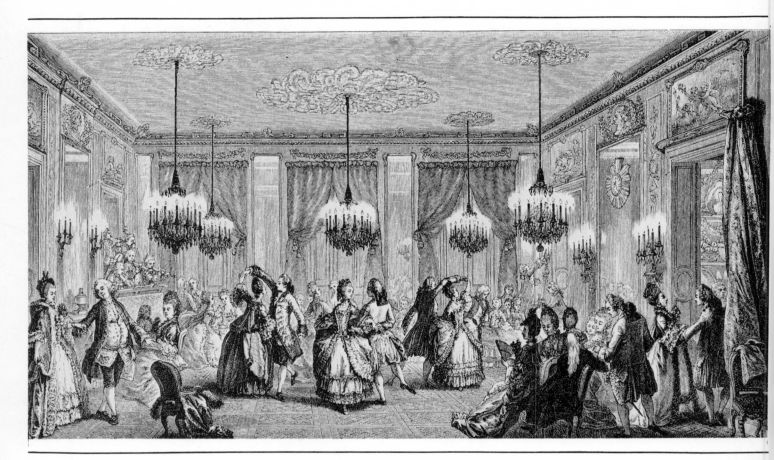

The restrained but intricate dancing that flourished in society's better homes during the eighteenth century. Decorum and quick feet were all-important.

*Men and women have always expressed socially
approved relations on the dance floor but the waltz was a
scandalous dance that shattered ballroom customs
stretching back to the court of Louis XIV.*

INTRODUCTION

No matter what the degree of proficiency involved, dancing is a factor in
virtually everyone's life. It is done at weddings, bar mitzvahs, and anniver-
saries, at special times like Christmas and the New Year, in schools, supper
clubs, and at those persistent "tea dance" get-togethers *(thés dansants)* which
are slowly making a comeback. It is especially popular on shipboard. Some
quit the floor at the first hint of a Latin rhythm, others dance all night, and
many indefatigable plodders do the fox-trot no matter what the music.
Whatever the case—it's a touch of dance fever.

Dancing is a highly visible, physical expression of social relations between men and women. Unwritten conventions that govern personal
conduct are demonstrated in the dances people do and the way they do
them. Dancing is fun, even intoxicating, but also a way of expressing
civilized behavior in a most pleasurable manner.

Moralists, watchdog commentators and social guardians from witch-hunter Cotton Mather to columnist Marya Mannes all keep a wary eye on the dance floor to see what people are dancing and to warn them when they have offended social propriety. Every generation has been chastised for "going too far," but the dances have continued to proliferate and still play an important role when men and women socialize.

Participational dancing has traditionally fallen into two patterns: that of the country, which we think of as folk, and that of the city, which we designate social. Both have existed as long as there have been town and country. They tend to follow their own lines of development but occasionally elements of one will cross over into the other and be absorbed quite happily.

The most proficient social dancers perform in exhibition competitions and then become teachers or coaches to other exhibition performers. Exhibition steps are always more glamorous than those that could be attempted on a crowded dance floor; they can be quite spectacular when seen on a big ballroom floor with acres of space. For the most part, regular social dancers are restricted by space and rein in their wilder impulses in the interest of mutual survival.

The element that stirs social arbiters' wrath is the close physical encounter that takes place on the dance floor. D.H. Lawrence, who spent a lifetime writing about love and its physical expression, referred to sex as the "dirty little secret" of Victorian society, and he, for one, let the secret out. His openness affected more than the literary world, and countless dancers were delighted to have the subject out in the open at last. Society tried to clamp the lid down on the obstreperous topic of sex but could no more do so than it could keep the waltz out of its ballrooms.

When the waltz first appeared it was considered absolutely scandalous. Today it seems the epitome of innocent and lighthearted diversion, the sort of activity that reflects propriety and wholesome sociability. It brings to mind salons and vast ballrooms, splendidly lit and decorated, filled with handsome, formally attired men partnering beautiful, elegantly turned out women, all swaying, turning, and gliding in an atmosphere of enchantment.

Well, the fuss concerned men and women embracing in public, for that is what the waltz required them to do openly, as it had never previously been done in social dancing. Although there had been varieties of social dance, all shared a common restraint which dictated that men and women dancing together could hold hands but should remain at arm's length. Partners also were to dance as part of a group of other couples and not go twirling off together, up to God knows what! Society was aware that dancing had a liberal dosage of sex laced into it, but no one was about to say so as long as that restraint prevailed. When the gap between partners closed, the pulpits thundered and commentators foresaw the collapse of civilization. As one homespun granny put it years later, "A dancing foot and a praying knee never grew on the same leg."

The dancing masters of the eighteenth and nineteenth centuries also saw a disregard for authority in the waltz. They saw individuals breaking away from the set patterns and formations of the minuet and schottische and a dozen other variants. In these, individuals were firmly merged into a social group and though partners might start and finish together, they frequently made exchanges during the course of the dance. There was little expression of individual choice; everything was regulated in accordance with the will of the dancing master who represented, at whatever remove, the ordered world of some royal court which had imposed its manners and ways on dancing. The dancing master was an important figure in court circles when it was expected that an aristocrat could dance, duel, and sit a horse properly. The nobility took instruction in all these diciplines and the dancing master regulated court entertainment in the name and by the authority of the king.

To defy these conventions meant, by implication, denying the social structure, letting a current of democracy waft into an autocratic society. The waltz, of course, didn't bring down the crowned heads of Europe; indeed, they ended up dancing it better than anyone else. However, the waltz was a highly visible symbol of changes that were taking place in society. But unlike other artistic expressions, it had no identifiable creator. It emerged in the countrysides of Austria and Germany without anyone claiming authorship, as is the pattern with most successful social dances in any era.

For the most part, anonymous dancers spontaneously create patterns of movement that are enjoyable and are also suitable to the mood of the time. Eventually dance teachers—not masters—come upon them and refine them into recognizable and repeatable patterns, give the resultant dance a name, and offer it for instruction.

These dances become little nuggets of social history to show us how people felt about themselves, one another, and their times. It was no accident that the unbridled twenties developed the exhibitionistic Charleston or the aggressive nineties the vigorous two-step. Neither could have emerged in the other's era, nor could the slinky togetherness of the Hustle, which is the expression of our own special dance fever.

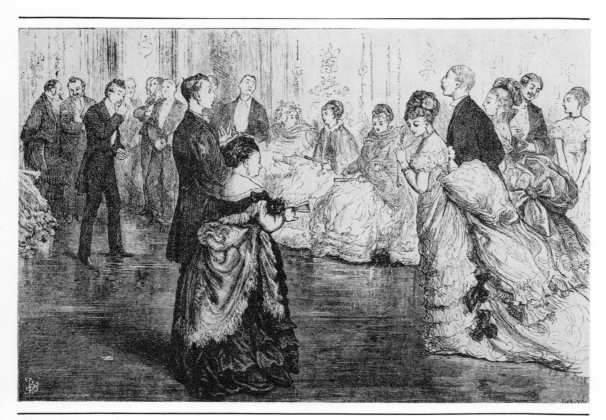

The first quadrille.

The Shakers seated men and women separately and kept them apart on the dance floor as well, in sharply defined formations.

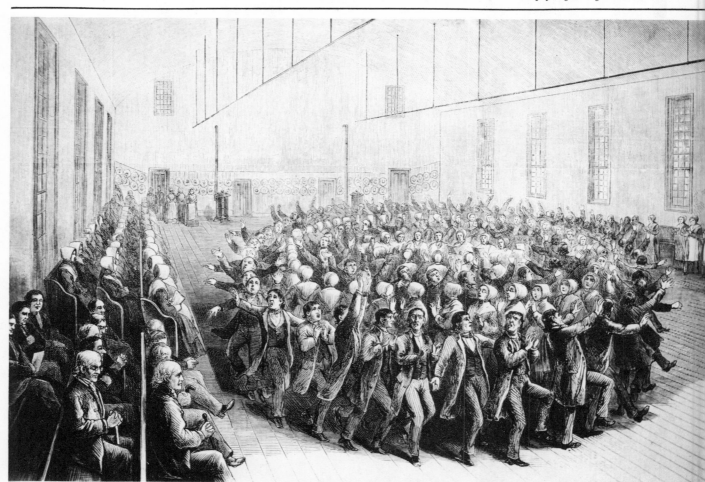

Puritans wouldn't dance on principle but other colonists did so eagerly. For the most part, though, they took European dances which were then modified to suit the country's special needs as people moved ever westward to the Pacific.

EARLY AMERICA DANCES

The only dancing in America when the Pilgram Fathers and Mothers landed was Indian religious ritual. The Puritans took a moral stand against dancing, so the country had to wait for other settlers before its social dance tradition could develop. In time they came, bringing with them their own native forms like the Irish jig, which eventually became tap dancing, and the statelier dances of European courts which were also modified. Those who worked the land and stayed in the countryside danced reels and fourhands and established the folk tradition. The Shakers, who were originally known as Shaking Quakers, danced to rid themselves of their sins. To be on the safe side, they saw to it that men and women remained absolutely separate and pounded around in penitential formations.

By the time of the Revolutionary War, the colonies had firmly established the boundaries between town and country. The seasonal ball was a great annual event held only in the cities. This ball was designated an "assembly" and the oldest of them, simply called The Assembly, was held in Philadelphia. It still is held there each year around Christmas time and is the direct descendant of the ones that George Washington attended. The Assembly put its best foot forward first in 1748; it was followed in 1762 by Charleston's St. Cecilia Society Ball. People were socially conscious to a degree and guests were invited according to social rank which was determined mainly by the size of the house they lived in.

The dances that the colonists favored were those which had been imported from England and had already been sanctioned at the formal balls there. These dances, like the minuet and the schottische, were danced at arm's length, and the whole of the evening was run under the watchful eye of a dancing master. He decided what would be danced and in what order and, in general, saw to it that the socially approved proprieties were maintained. Young men and young women as well as gentlemen and ladies went for regular dance instruction. George Washington is known to have written a letter intended to make sure that his nephew was properly instructed. Dancing was a social grace that one had to acquire in order to be accepted in the eighteenth century. Discipline in dancing fostered discipline in society, or so it was felt. In our own time, the late William De Rham, New York society's premier dancing teacher, sternly warned little boys not to abandon their female partners until the latter acquired another partner or got married! Social dancing may have looked like simple fun but it quietly instilled a sense of order and correct behavior between the sexes as well.

The American population rolled steadily westward, dancing all the way. By the time it reached the California coast, the Wagon Wheel, the Texas Star, and the Arkansas Traveler had become popular dances, among others, and their spirit was slowly but surely changing the European dance forms that had been inherited earlier. Americans performed the traditional dances with a great sense of freedom. The minuet had flourished at the French court and in its time represented a high point of complexity in

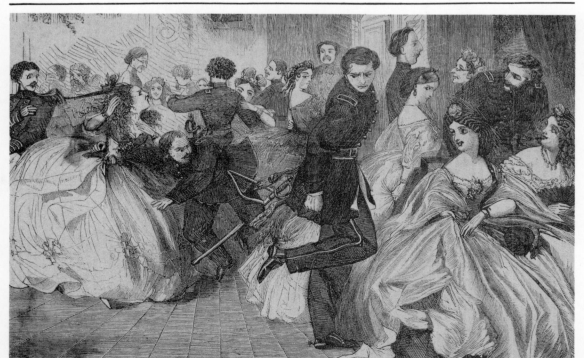

Spurs, swords, and epaulettes wage their own war on crinoline at a military ball.

the tradition of social dancing. When it reached America, it was slowed down to a gliding walk and became the quadrille that was so popular in the South. The schottische, in England, was referred to as a German polka and here was danced in a less frenzied fashion. But, though Americans changed the ways in which dancing was performed, they were still dependent on Europe for the basic forms of the social dances.

The sense of reserve and order that were imbedded in the European dance forms were reflected in the American ones as well. The concept of a couple as an independent entity did not exist. People danced together as groups and the group sense was expressed in square dancing as well as the more restrained dancing in the cities. Frontier women worked alongside their men to a greater extent than did their city sisters and, as a result, the dancing they did reflected a more comradely sense of sharing.

The polka, which spread through Europe in the middle of the nineteenth century, received its name from the Bohemian word *pulka* which means half. It described the short half-step that is characteristic of the dance and the polka was taken up in both city ballrooms and country dancing. Generally though, city dwellers and country folk kept to themselves socially, developing their own distinctive patterns of culture. The caller who chanted the sequence of steps, maintained order in the country and the dancing master ruled the roost in the city.

The Civil War stimulated the industrialization of the country which continued at full throttle though hampered by periodic "panics" and "crashes." In the West, great cattle drives supplied meat for the tables of the East, and Eastern bankers steadily pushed the railroad westward. Fortunes were made and lost midst the restless activity. An eager press covered developments with a hunger for the sensational and sometimes with investigative energy. The papers themselves competed fiercely for readers and mounted extravagant efforts to attract them. In 1871 *The New York Herald* sent its reporter Henry M. Stanley to the African continent with instructions to find the lost Scottish missionary Dr. David Livingstone. He did, and greeted the astonished cleric with the immortal understatement, "Dr. Livingstone, I presume."

While the East industrialized, the West was still forming itself into states to join the Union. On April 22, 1889, when the Oklahoma Territory was opened for settlement, 15,000 people crossed the line of demarcation to enter the Territory and file land claims that same day. A year later, Joseph Pulitzer publisher of *The New York World,* sent his reporter Elizabeth Corcoran to circumnavigate the globe. She achieved fame as "Nelly Bly" and by making the trip in 72 days, 6 hours, 11 minutes, and 14 seconds, demolished the 80-day record logged by the fictional Phineas Fogg. She was immortalized in the song commemorating her feat.

The energy of the country generated wealth which became concentrated in the hands of a few. These privileged few lived extraordinarily well, built enormous mansions to reside in during the winter and lavish seaside and country "cottages" to vacation in during the summer. They entertained on a royal scale and they danced in glorious surroundings.

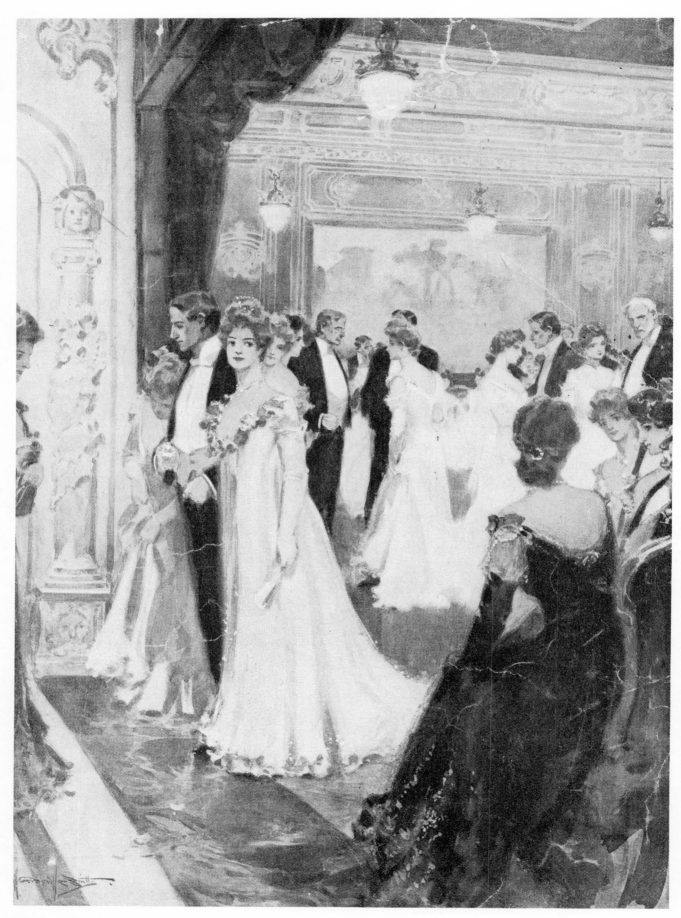

The ballroom of the William C. Whitney mansion.

*Enormous wealth created society's Four Hundred
and rank, very definitely, had its privileges.
Women blossomed at balls where the waltz and the two-step
predominated and Harriet Hubbard Ayer wrote a health and
beauty column for young women in which she quite
openly advocated the discreet use of cosmetics.*

THREE QUARTER TIME AND SOUSA MARCHES

The stylishly dressed woman of the gay nineties had only recently escaped from the bulky bustle which had made her appear like the front end of a short sofa. She was still bundled up to the chin but had very definitely transferred the emphasis from the "lower back" to the upper torso and in particular the shoulders. Sleeves grew to enormous sizes and blouses, dresses, and coats conspicuously consumed yards and yards of material. Hems still dipped down to the ground and feet remained discreetly hidden. The well dressed woman's gloves sported long, time-consuming rows of buttons, as did her shoes that had to be laboriously fastened with a buttonhook.

The modish waist was very tight, the collar very high, and the corset almost impregnable. The fashionable woman tied herself, or had herself tied, into fashion with a deep breath and the help of drawstrings that tightened her foundation garment to a degree that jeopardized her health.

Actual cases of internal organ displacement were known. She piled her hair high on her head in elaborately staged bundles and then perched tiny hats precariously on top of the coiffure. In the winter she completed the ensemble with a large muff. It seems almost a miracle that any of these women survived. But they not only survived, they danced, and very adroitly.

The favorite dances of the gay nineties were the waltz and the two-step. The latter was related to a march step. John Philip Sousa made a fortune for himself and his band writing full-blooded marches: he introduced "The Washington Post" in 1891 and at the end of the decade capped this success with the immensely popular "Stars and Stripes Forever." He was a martinet of a conductor and retained his military bearing even after he had resigned as leader of the United States Marine Corps Band. The country couldn't get enough of Sousa and his marches and positively galloped along in step to their spritely cadences.

Sousa commented bluntly that a good march should make even a man with a wooden leg "step out." It was robust music and thoroughly consistent with the country's belligerent posture toward its neighbors. Colonel Theodore (Teddy) Roosevelt led his Rough Riders up the slopes of San Juan Hill in Cuba during the Spanish-American War, and halfway around the world Admiral George Dewey won the battle of Manila Bay by beating the Spanish Pacific fleet there. The war, which had begun in the spring, ended in December and the United States acquired from it an offshore empire in the Caribbean and the Pacific as well as a reputation as an international power. In spirit and tempo Sousa's marches were decidedly apt.

On the lighter side of life, Americans rolled joyously along on the redesigned bicycle with comfortable pneumatic tires. The older big-wheel style was replaced by a model with a pair of identically sized soft wheels that allowed women to take gracefully to the roads. They did so enthusiastically. What had been a strenuously athletic balancing act on the old contraption became a delightful social activity on the new. Hefty Diamond Jim Brady who didn't like to ride, gave a gold-plated bicycle to his adored Lillian Russell to help her lose a little weight by pedaling through New York's Central Park.

Young men and women wheeled off on picnics and sightseeing trips and bicycle repair shops proliferated. Two young men in Ohio, Orville and Wilbur Wright, supported themselves repairing these machines while thinking ahead to a more dramatic form of transportation, and Henry Ford built his first automobile. Gold was discovered in the Klondike region and set off a rush to Alaska, and pianist Ben Harney set off another rush when he introduced ragtime to the patrons of Tony Pastor's garden restaurant in New York. But that came toward the end of the decade. For most of the nineties, people danced quickly to Sousa's marches and more flowingly to the waltz. The latter was the sentimental favorite by far of a sentimental age, and no one expressed the fact more eloquently than Charles K. Harris who wrote "After the Ball."

The dramatic situation the song described was improbable, but it expressed the slushy pieties of the day exquisitely. A man abandoned his ballroom companion without a word after he saw her kissing another. He didn't know at the time that it was her brother and so as an old man, still a bachelor, he melodiously regrets his precipitous action. Harris, who later set up a song writing school to teach others the secret of his success, became a rich man from this song.

Before the decade was out, song writers had produced "She's Only a Bird in a Gilded Cage," "The Band Played On," "When You were Sweet Sixteen," "America the Beautiful," "The Sidewalks of New York," and "Ta-ra-ra-boom-deay." The last had its rowdy origin in a St. Louis brothel where the girls used to do a particularly intriguing dance while singing it. Of course, the public would have been shocked, but then the public wasn't told where the tune came from any more than it was aware that the ragtime lilt, beginning to make its impact, was New Orleans saloon and whorehouse music. Concurrently, Mildred J. Hill, a schoolteacher, wrote a little song for her class called "Good Morning to You" which achieved universal fame as "Happy Birthday to You."

Since there were no radios and phonographs were in their expensive infancy, people danced to the sound of live music. They danced most elegantly at the great hotels, opera-house galas, and balls in private homes. Among the formidable society matrons, none was more imperious than Mrs. Cornelius Vanderbilt II whose social advisor and confidant was newspaperman Ward McAllister. His power was assured by the relationship, and his columns had the authority of scripture. With a stroke of the pen he created the most copied elite of the day: the Four Hundred. These were the most enviable—or at least envied—people in the country and there were four hundred of them because that was the capacity of Alice Vanderbilt's ballroom in her Fifth Avenue mansion. And when they gathered, they waltzed.

In the classic waltz position, the man faced his partner, placed his right arm around her waist, and grasped her extended right hand with his left; she delicately posed her left hand on his shoulder. There was normally a space between the two that widened or narrowed depending on the mood of the moment. The pair turned round and round and toured the hall as part of swaying circles of other dancers doing the same thing. The total image was that of swirling, fast-moving crowds of couples, each dancer locked into his or her partner's embrace and gaze. The stiffness of the older, set dances, with their measured cadences, had vanished. Couples no longer looked to a dancing master to take their cues; they looked in one another's eyes, which kept them from becoming dizzy, and effectively blocked out the rest of the world. No wonder the older dancing masters had seen the waltz as a menace! Couples had eyes only for one another and not for the authority of society's delegated representative, the dancing master.

The elaborately staged balls were the most important social events of the season. It was necessary to see others and to be seen; women carried

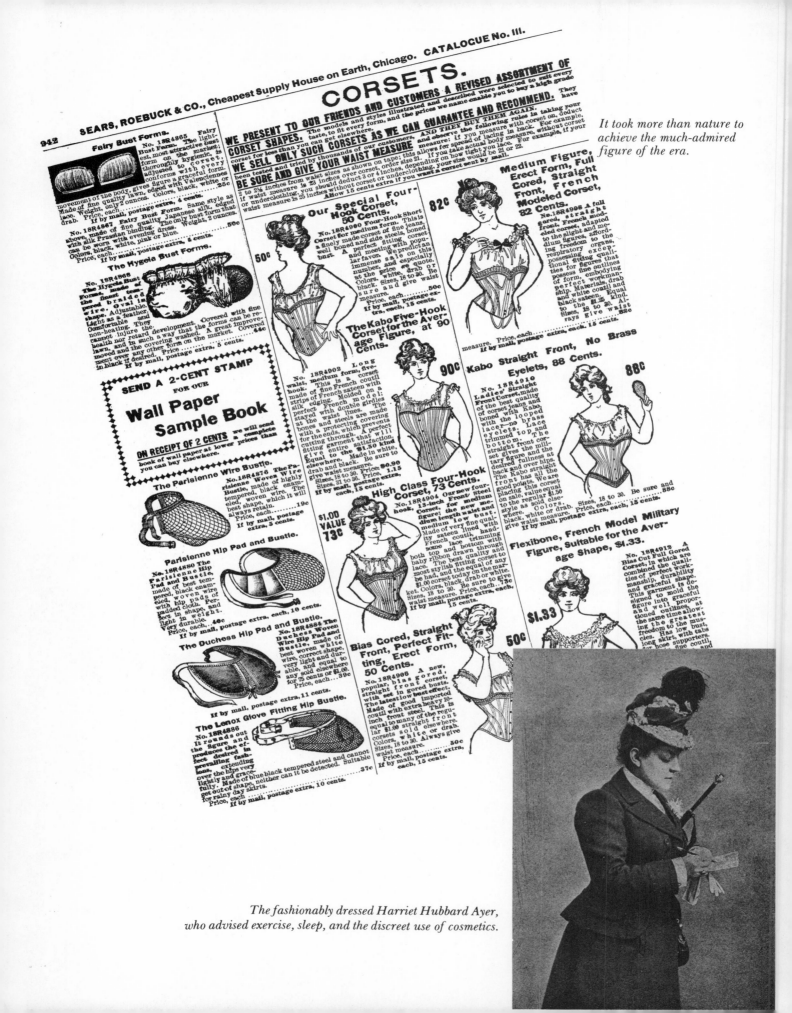

It took more than nature to achieve the much-admired figure of the era.

The fashionably dressed Harriet Hubbard Ayer, who advised exercise, sleep, and the discreet use of cosmetics.

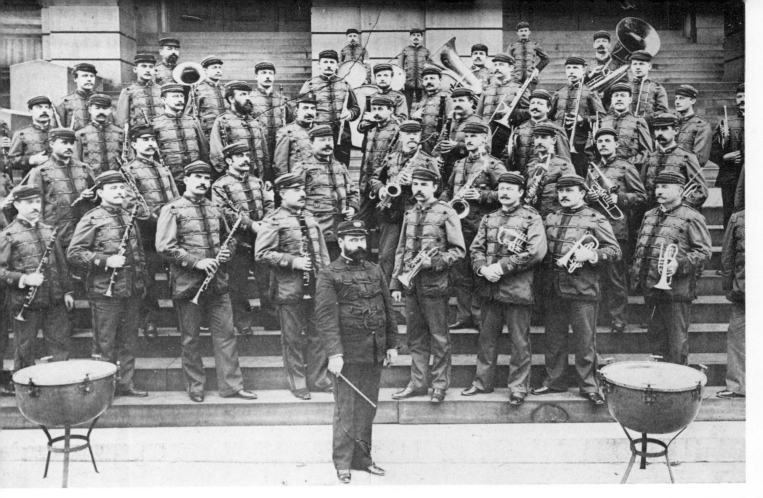

The march king John Philip Sousa and band.

The Columbian Ball at Madison Square Garden where gentlemen's arms circled ladies' waists unashamedly.

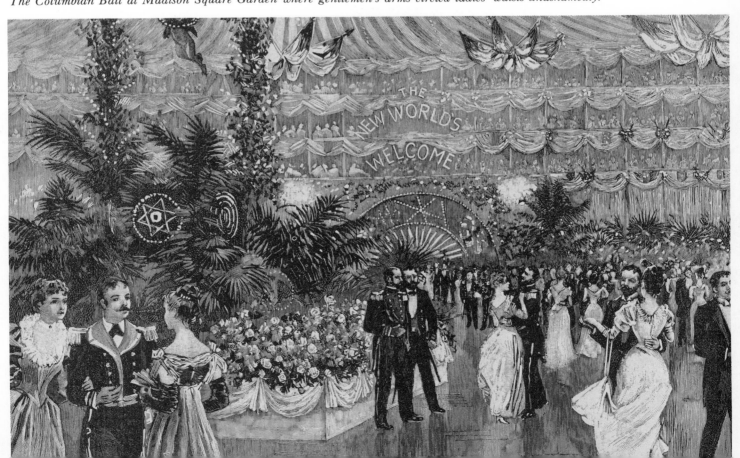

beautiful *carnets de bal,* which had to be filled, if only to compare with others'. These dance cards were affixed to the wrist or enclosed in expensive and elaborate cases; in many instances they were chased with gold and decorated with gemstones. A tiny gold pencil enabled a gentleman to inscribe his name in the numbered space that showed the dance that had been allotted to him. The whole thing was ritual; it was romance, and it was socially sanctioned amidst elaborate rules of behavior. No gentleman was expected to monopolize the whole dance card even though he might have wanted to. No lady was expected to allow a gentleman the liberty of more than a proper share of her time unless, of course, they were formally pledged. The rules of the dance floor were as baroque as the architecture of the buildings in which they were enacted. Rules and order prevailed, governing the numbers of dances and the proper distance between partners, but these were rearguard actions of a society that had already made the biggest capitulation of all by endorsing the waltz. Once those couples had embraced in full public view, it would be impossible to separate them into regimented squadrons again, drilling away under the watchful eyes of a dancing master. Society could still be shocked at reckless dancing or too close an embrace, but after the waltz gained entry there was no turning back to arm's length dancing.

This contemporary account of the ball is couched in terms of delicate understatement but the author's drift is clear. "Many and mixed are the motives which attract the pleasure seeker to the ball, but over an assemblage of youth and beauty, Dan Cupid shoots his feathery darts broadcast, and though he may not hit the heart he aims for, he generally has occasion to exult next day over a large and varied collection of trophies: broken fans, lost gloves, diamond engagement rings, bits of torn lace, faded bouquets and soiled orders of dancing, and—let us hope not very often—a broken heart or two in the bargain."

To prepare for the ball, women not only had to dress themselves and their hair, they had to make certain basic decisions about what cosmetic help would be permissible. Cosmetics had been around as long as recorded history. Ancient Egyptian women used green eye shadow and in the Far East nightingale dung was highly prized as a coloring agent. However the gay nineties looked upon cosmetics with some suspicion. The climate was changing but there was a feeling that only women of a certain sort used cosmetics and they were either *demimondaines* or "advanced." Fortunately, Harriet Hubbard Ayer was neither. She was a well-traveled, educated, society woman who had to earn a living after her divorce. She put out a jar of face cream which she said she discovered in Paris and was based on the same formula as that used by the celebrated French beauty Madame Récamier. Mrs. Ayer had a social reputation and a marketing sense that any businessman of the day would have been proud of. She advertised cleverly and built up the first great cosmetic house in the United States. By 1896 she was contributing a weekly column to *The New York World,* advising young women on health and beauty. She stressed the health aspect of the cosmetics and made plain good sense in her advocacy of rest, bathing, and fresh air. She gave formulas for preparations that would help the complexion and rid the face of wrinkles, and, of course, she didn't fail to promote her own line of products. All this was a far cry from the surreptitious use of burnt cork for eyelashes and of rice powder to achieve the "interesting" pale look then in fashion. Mrs. Ayer discouraged the feminine image of the frail, shrinking flower and positively scorned dowdiness, labeling it a sin.

Still, it was a courageous young woman who used rouge, which was like a red flag for attracting social disapproval. Mrs. Ayer refused to listen to the disapprovers and set down some commonsense rules governing the use of cosmetics which she felt were justified. Basically, she said over and over, it was really up to the woman herself to decide, the time of decision being age thirty. Younger than that she didn't think cosmetics were really necessary, except in rare cases, though she did leave an opening for those who attended balls and opera galas. There cosmetics could be considered a necessity to protect oneself from the dazzling light of electricity as contrasted with the softer glow of candlelight. She referred to cosmetics humorously as "war paint," and always advised that they be used discreetly, especially in the daytime.

Outside of the ballroom, life went on. In Chicago the first all-steel frame building was erected and the inventor W. L. Judson developed the zipper. Murray Teichman was born on the Lower East Side of New York; he was to create a mail-order home instructional manual for dancers and call himself Arthur Murray. Dave Genaro and Ray Bailey popularized the cake walk, an old minstrel show dance, in the hit show *Rastus on Parade*. King C. Gillette removed some of the adventure from the morning shaving ritual by patenting the safety razor. Just before the bells of the new century pealed, song writer Paul Dresser, social novelist Theodore Dreiser's brother, published "On the Banks of the Wabash." The folks back home in Indiana made it the state's official song and everyone looked ahead optimistically, wondering what the new century had in store.

A roofgarden restaurant in New York with the band and dance floor at the rear.

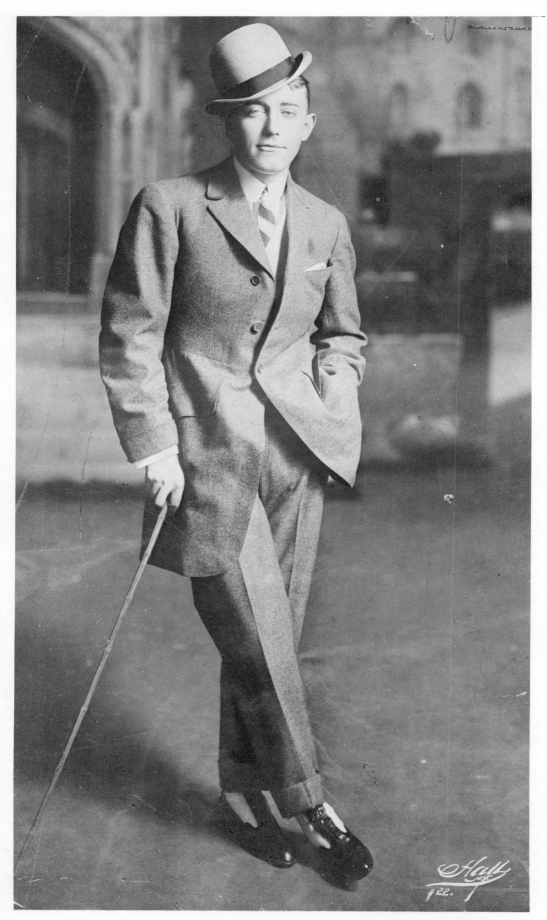

The Yankee Doodle Boy himself, George M. Cohan.

Exuberance fairly burst out of the country's new president "Teddy" Roosevelt. Ragtime music accompanied a flock of energetic new dances and the Wright brothers proved that man could fly. The country was excited and enthusiastic about all the new possibilities.

QUICK STEP

The optimism of a prospering nation at the start of a new century was understandable enough, and six pretty girls captured the innocent mood in "Florodora." The sextet "Tell Me Pretty Maiden Are There Any More at Home Like You?" saw handsome young gentlemen in top hats paying musical court to frilly and picture-hatted young ladies. It was startling to remember that a hundred years before the country had barely concluded a successful colonial revolt; it was now an imperial power with its own colonies.

William McKinley was elected president in 1897 and Teddy Roosevelt was his vice-president. Four years later, after McKinley had been assassinated, Roosevelt, at forty-two, became the youngest president in history. His six children's laughter and his own dynamic roar filled the White House with liveliness. He was an outdoorsman, a patrician of Dutch ancestry, a successful soldier, an avid reader, and, in foreign policy, he carried a "big stick."

During Roosevelt's presidency, the Panama Canal was completed, the first great national parks were established, and the Pure Food and Drug Act was passed to regulate an industry that was then dangerously uncontrolled. T.R. went after monopolistic practices in businesses and also found time to put a needy poet on the federal payroll in New York. Later, Edwin Arlington Robinson would win the Pulitzer Prize for his verse. Teddy was just right for the times. He was brash, sentimental, hardheaded; he kept a sense of fair play and his zest for life reflected the feelings of the country.

The Florodora girls were living examples of an idealized type of feminine beauty that had been categorized as the Gibson girl. Her hair was piled up casually on top of her head and she had a faintly haughty air. She looked very capable and yet was modest in her dress, suggesting a flavor of the previous century. Charles Dana Gibson, the best-known illustrator of his time, had created an ideal for the American woman. Teddy's eldest daughter Alice was a perfect example and set tongues wagging with her devil-take-the-hindmost air. She danced till dawn and quite often let her dance card be monopolized by young gentlemen whom she might more diplomatically have avoided. T.R. muttered that she hardly ever rose before noon because of her late hours, but he didn't clamp the lid on her social life. Times were changing indeed.

In society gatherings they still danced the waltz and the two-step as well as the polka and an occasional schottische. The more raffish elements capered about in bordellos and various "sporting" districts doing dances that had not yet made their appearence in polite society. They were like the locals in Austria, in country inns and taverns over a century earlier who gave the waltz to the world. Inevitably, what started in New Orleans slowly spread throughout the nation.

Two names dominated the musical stage, Victor Herbert and George M. Cohan. Both were Irish; Herbert was even born on the other side. Both expressed the energy and vitality of America in tunes that everyone knew.

Herbert was a classically trained musician who wrote in the operetta tradition. By the end of the decade he had composed a love song to his adopted city, "In Old New York," and celebrated beautiful women with a bouquet of songs: "Everyday Is Ladies' Day for Me," "Kiss Me Again," "Ah Sweet Mystery of Life," and "I'm Falling In Love with Someone."

Cohan, a stage trouper from childhood who wore his heart on his sleeve, wrote "Give My Regards to Broadway," "The Yankee Doodle Boy," "Mary," and "You're a Grand Old Flag." Both men alternately captured the theater audiences' hearts as the country itself was swayed now by the appeal of the settled era just past, now by the enticing possibilities of the first decade of a new century.

Moving to the foreground was a new syncopated sound that anticipated or delayed natural accents in music and shifted them to "off" beats; it was called ragtime. It ushered in a world of new and scandalous dances that appalled the more conservative elements of society. It was as if a zoo had suddenly opened up on the dance floor with the Grizzly Bear, the Bunny-Hug, the Turkey-Trot, the Kangaroo Dip, the Horse-Trot, and the

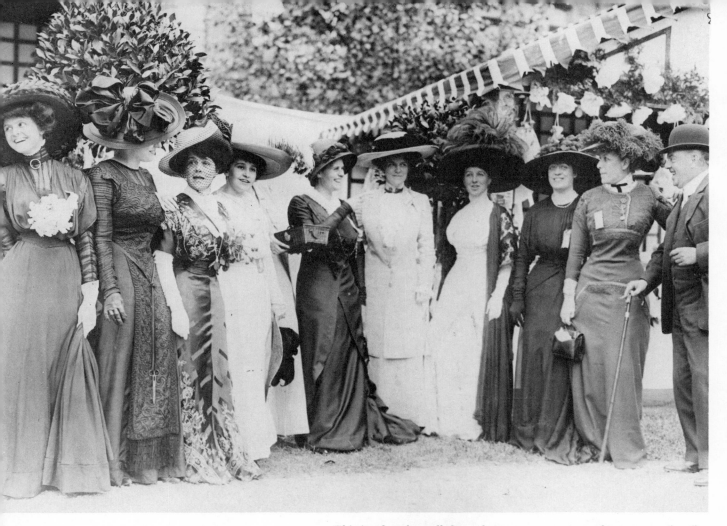

This is what the well-dressed woman wore at an afternoon garden fête.

Snake. The dances all had one thing in common: the boys and girls were closer together than ever before and they weren't standing solidly on their own two feet. The young lady clung, perilously off balance, to the young gentleman, either locking her arms around his neck or leaning back, completely supported by his manly strength. Together they went prancing along at a rapid, energetic pace like the decade itself.

Women were beginning to dress a bit more aggressively as they began to emerge from the protective Victorian proprieties that had encased them as tightly as their corsets. The S shape for the female body was now in order, though with the emphasis on the bust rather than the hips. American clothes designers, so long in thrall to what was happening in Paris, introduced the shirtwaist, a simple blouse to be tucked into a skirt. It became the rage. Sleeves, which had been puffed out beyond reason, began to shrink in diameter and waistlines became a bit more sensible and natural. Skirts still brushed the floor but were not quite so voluminous and women bought more and more ready-to-wear clothes. Toward the end of the decade, the waistline was moved higher and the dresses themselves became more sculptured and flowing.

Hair was still piled on top of the head but was tipped forward more aggressively; the silly little hats of the gay nineties were banished. They were replaced by enormous feathered creations, the demand for which

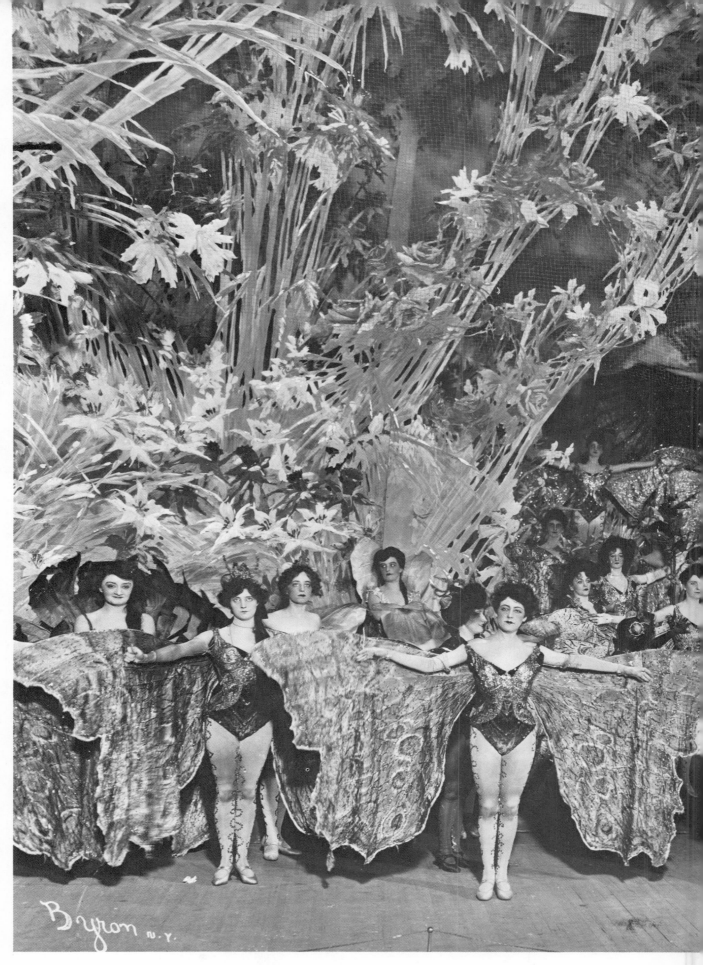

Tableau from Victor Herbert's Babes In Toyland.

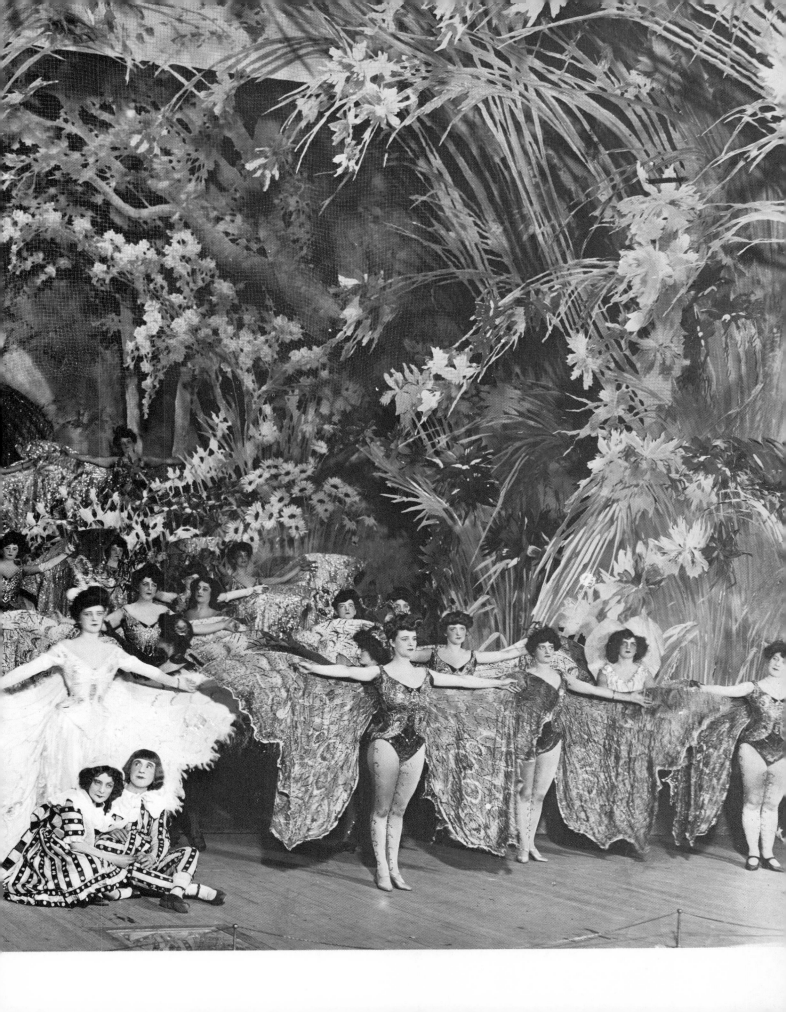

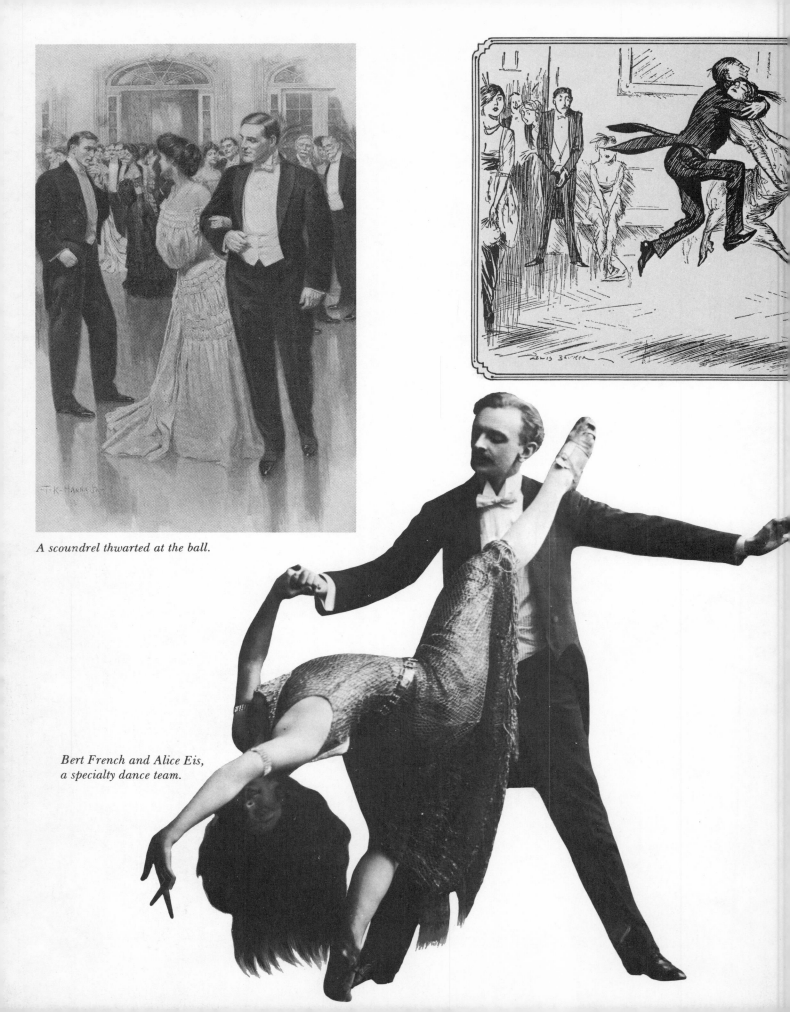

A scoundrel thwarted at the ball.

Bert French and Alice Eis,
a specialty dance team.

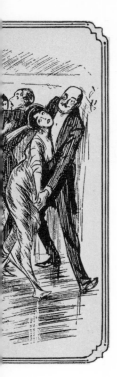

A cartoonist's rendering of the latest fad dance.

threatened to wipe out the bird population of several continents before it abated. Finally those pretty ecological disasters were replaced by broad-brimmed "picture" hats which were just as flattering and far easier on wildlife.

Lotions and creams were used to a greater and greater degree as beauty aids. The most outrageous frauds among them were abolished only after passage of the Pure Food and Drug Act in 1906. Still, the idea that beauty aids might be used without incurring social ostracism had arrived. It wasn't yet quite nice to color one's hair, but then that was looked at askance even fifty years later.

Decorum could still be relied upon to keep the dance floors of the rich in order, and it did for the most part in the major balls in New York and such lush watering spots as Saratoga and Newport. But as the decade wore on, ragtime dictated dance time to a greater and greater extent. As ragtime took hold, the first uninhibited dance craze began. The chief offender was the Turkey-Trot which even drew disapproval from the Vatican for its grotesque gyrations. Actually, a room full of bobbing and ducking couples might be regarded as funny, but society cast a disapproving glance at couples clasped together doing a deep dip forward and repeating the same thing to the rear, or doing fancy leg-crossing steps as they swiveled away from and toward one another. The waltz, in which people embraced, was risky enough but this was positively athletic and it wasn't a smooth gliding in three-quarter time; it was weaving and swaying to two-four meter.

On this occasion at least, the more traditional dances predominate.

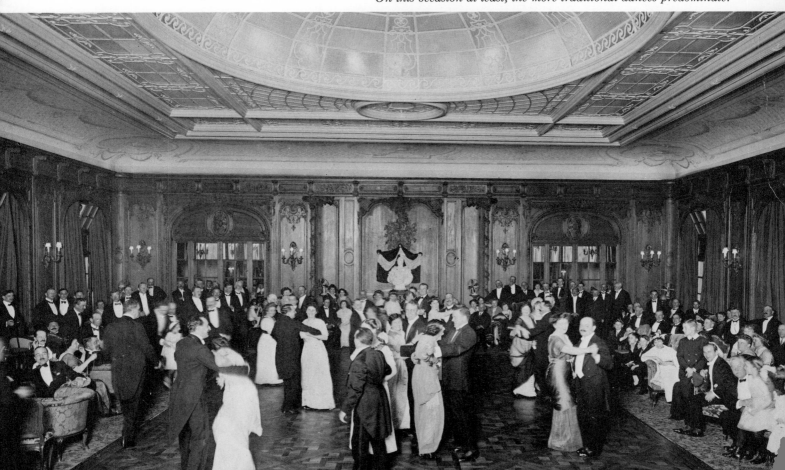

If society's watchdogs frowned on the Turkey-Trot, they became near apoplectic over the Grizzly Bear which was known in some quarters as the Texas Tommy. It didn't sway, it swooped, and a rocking aggressiveness made it an ideal subject for cartoonists. Women appeared to be hanging on to their partners for dear life and the men looked like frenzied primates. There were two basic positions for the dance and partners used both during the course of a good set. The man clasped his partner around the waist with his left arm and supported the back of her head with his right. His partner slung one arm over his left shoulder and around his neck while slipping the other one up to the middle of his back. She was as secure as a koala cub. The other basic position was a slight variant of this: his left arm still circled her waist but his right arm was over her shoulder and around her neck. She responded by hooking her arms on his shoulders as if she were preparing to do chin-ups. Thus locked, a couple was launched on to the dance floor in a tussling mass. A quick eight-count jog forward was halted with a roller coaster sway, followed by a similar series of steps with a bent-knee dip. Couples could move to the right or to the left but stayed as close as two peas in a pod.

The young lady who enjoyed such dancing had a degree of freedom that had not been possible on the dance floor in the previous century, but she was still severely discriminated against in the world of politics and property. In one out of four states the married woman couldn't legally own property and in a third of the states she had no claim on her own earnings. The fact that she was allowed to have earnings at all was a small triumph, but old customs died hard and to a great extent there was no real career for a woman outside marriage.

The invention of a practical typewriter and its obvious advantage over handwriting opened career doors in a way that nothing before it had done. Men either couldn't or more likely wouldn't learn to operate the newfang-

Proms have always meant dancing.

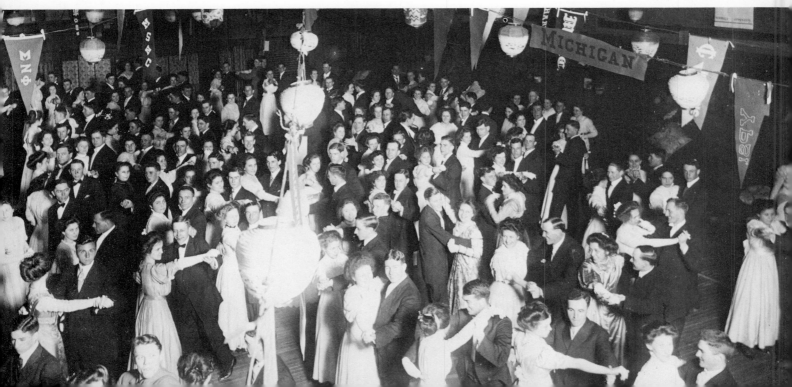

led things that were so much more efficient and legible than script, but women had no qualms at all about learning if it meant the possibility of office work. The salaries offered were so much better than the money to be earned from cleaning and washing; the work also brought women into honorable contact with eligible young men. Shirtwaists seemed just the ideal sort of outfit for the emerging businesswoman.

The decade tossed restlessly back and forth between the stability of the recent past and the excitement of the future. The Wright brothers made the first powered flight in 1903 and though it lasted under a minute, the exploration of the sky had begun. Only the year before, a contented country had been humming "In the Good Old Summertime." In 1904 the St. Louis Exposition caught everyone's attention. Almost immediately "Meet Me in St. Louis" detailed the plight of a young husband returning home to find that his bride had left him for the bright lights in St. Louis and now invited him (Louie) to meet her in St. Louis if he wanted to see her again.

The next year a song plaintively inquired "Will You Love Me in December As You Do in May?" The words were written by Jimmy Walker who was later to become mayor of New York, acquire a reputation as a ladies' man, and be driven into exile by a bluenosed reform movement. A few years later the man's side of the coin was portrayed in "I Wonder Who's Kissing Her Now."

The unrest that started in the gay nineties was budding but it had not yet blossomed. Social restraints were still powerful enough to slow down the pace of the change. Men were allowed to wear something resembling a sensible bathing suit but women's cumbrous bathing attire (hats, skirts, stockings and shoes) made it hazardous for them to do anything more daring than get their knees damp. (They *did* begin to play tennis). Although the populations of the big cities were just touching the million mark, three-fifths of the country still lived in small towns, and small towns were not quite ready for the new woman. There was nothing, however, that could stop technical progress and each invention opened career possibilities for women as well as men.

The Great Train Robery was the first real movie and it was shown in 1903, a time when the bicycle was still going strong and the automobile had begun to make its entrance. The automobile was faster than the bicycle, the plane was more exciting than either, and the dances became wilder and wilder. The sound of ragtime ruled an ever-widening circle of dance floors. It slipped out of the red light districts right into college proms. Anarchy appeared to be taking over the social dance.

If waltzing couples were mindful only of one another, the Grizzly Bear fanciers were heedless of life and limb; but there was no denying the appeal of these hug-and-tussle dances. Partners danced cheek to cheek, with "lower backs" provocatively thrust out. The smooth-gliding nineties were being left further and further behind, though the public was humming "Put On Your Old Grey Bonnet" as the decade slipped away and had taken time out to establish Mother's Day.

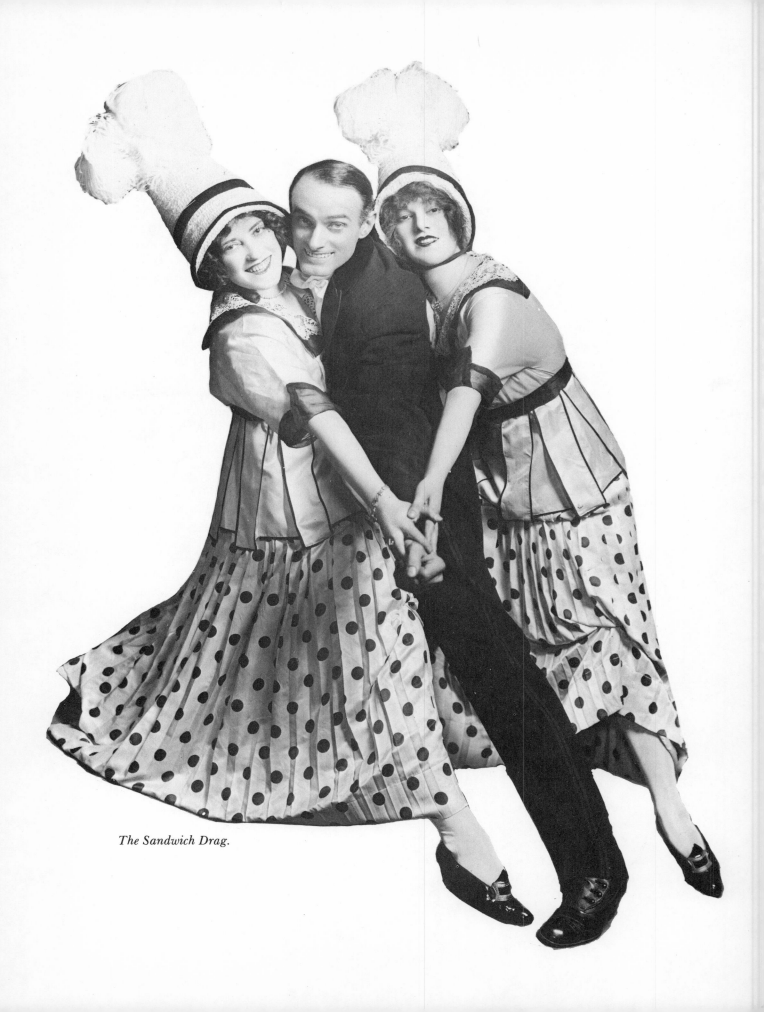

The Sandwich Drag.

1910-1919

*Vernon and Irene Castle showed that the raucous
new dances could also be performed with grace and elegance
but Boston banned the tango anyway. World War I cast a harsh
shadow across the land and also accelerated the social changes
that were bringing women out into the world.*

RAGTIME

The new dance craze had gone much too far in the eyes of people charged
with sponsoring charity balls. Many social patrons began to cancel some of
the events rather than have them profaned by the outlandish new dances.
Whether organizers chose to suppress or cancel, they were shocked. A
reporter from *The Sun* spoke to Mrs. Arthur M. Dodge, one of the organizers of a fashionable annual ball, the New York Junior Cotillion. "The
real tango, I am told, by those who have seen it danced in Argentina and
elsewhere, would never be permitted, even in the variety theater in New
York, and *that* is saying a great deal," she huffed.

If Mrs. Dodge felt that way about the tango, Mae Holstead Beatty, the
inspector appointed by the New York Board of Education to evaluate its
social program, felt that way about the whole menagerie of dances that had
been turned loose. Prior to the First World War, the city maintained school
recreation centers at which dancing was a very popular pastime. Just to

make sure that nothing untoward happened there in the course of an evening, they sent Miss Beatty around to the centers in fifty-eight public schools to prepare a report. To quote Miss Beatty, "I have surveyed the field thoroughly, prior to handing in my report and believe this is the wisest plan for us. You know perfectly well that these dances came to us from the Barbary Coast, the apaches of Paris and similar other untutored sources. The movements of various dances assisted by the music to which they are danced stimulate too much abandon, too much swaggering, too much freedom . . . so we will stick to the twostep, the waltz and the quadrille as formerly we've danced them."

Miss Beatty may have been a bit of a prude but she was right on target in spotting the sources of the dances. They certainly did not originate at the highest levels of society; but then popular dancing never does. They did come out of "sporting" districts and there was nothing that could be done to keep them there. The public liked them. Other public institutions tried a different tack and imported dancers from Castle House in Manhattan to teach the younger generation a more refined version of the rowdy dances. The goal in effect, was to teach them to dance the way Vernon and Irene Castle did.

The Castles on a dance floor were everything society considered elegant and sophisticated. When Irene wore a headband across her brow, it became instantly fashionable as the Castleband. When they did the maxixe (pronounced mashish) and the tango, it became imperative to be able to dance them as the Castles did. The couple dominated the decade until Vernon was killed in an air crash in 1918. They were the most acclaimed dancing partners of the time and twenty years later, inevitably, Fred Astaire and Ginger Rogers turned their saga into a successful film, *The Story of Vernon and Irene Castle*.

Vernon (Blyth) was English and Irene (Foote) was American. They first gained renown in France doing a nightclub act at the fashionable Café de Paris. They had married in 1911 and after minor roles in the theater decided that exhibition dancing in Paris would be a welcome change. Irene didn't even have an evening dress, so she wore her wedding gown the first time they appeared. Before long, as infatuated patrons pressed money on her and her partner to demonstrate a special number, she wore the finest in high fashion. At one after-hours party she and Vernon clowned around with a one-step and changed the accent of the movement. "We went up when the beat went down," Irene later explained about the casual invention of the Castle Walk.

The Castles did a number of things that were different, but the chief ingredient in all their experimentation was an air of cool elegance that was in complete contrast to the wrestling of the Turkey-Trot and its ilk. They declared war on the menagerie dances by the example of their own exhibition dancing and through teaching, in private lessons, at $100 an hour to the rich and at a considerably cheaper rate to the less advantaged. Boston simply banned the tango in a fit of pique but then Boston had also banned croquet. The Castles performed the tango stylishly and with restraint. They took one step forward, slid the second foot up and to the side, and brought the first foot over to it. The initial steps were done quickly and the closing step slowly. The close could be delayed by adding several more forward steps and then bringing the feet together. The Castles dipped, promenaded, rocked, and checked to this enchanting rhythm and the public began to favor their more sophisticated rendition of the tango. They popularized the Hesitation Waltz, the Castle Walk of course and the maxixe which was also referred to as the Brazilian tango. When Vernon died, Irene retired, but by that time most of the beast dances were back in their cages or at least performing like well brought up turkeys, grizzlies, bunnies, and snakes.

In the previous decade, dancing had begun to spread from private homes into hotels and cabarets and the Castles gave it a push with the creation of late afternoon dancing parties called *thés dansants.* Young men and women flocked to the restaurants and hotels, which featured a little food and a lot of dancing. Dancing became of the utmost importance to song publishers who had to feed the insatiable public appetite for suitable music and they insisted that their writers produce danceable tunes. A Broadway performer, Harry Fox, improvised a little dance in 1913 while appearing in the Ziegfeld Follies and when slowed a bit by teacher Oscar Duryea, it caught on as the fox-trot. Out of this minor improvisation was born the single most popular dance in social dance history. It was a combination of the old marching step and the new ragtime syncopation. Mr. Fox's step swept the dancing world and music publishers translated much of their material into its four-quarter cadences.

There was another madness abroad, in addition to dance fever, and it erupted into World War I as Europe mobilized for the grimmest war of modern times. Armies were mired in opposing trenches from France across Holland to the North Sea. Typhus killed thousands there—adding to the more than 20 million people around the globe carried off by influenza before the end of the decade. Three-quarters of a million soldiers were killed or wounded fighting over a few miles of territory at Verdun. Unseen, submarines sent ships to the bottom and from the air, bombs were dropped on civilians as well as soldiers. The world definitely had broken with the pieties of a bygone age.

At the beginning of the decade, intoxicated with the new accomplishment of flying, Americans sang "Come Josephine in My Flying Machine" but soon were singing angrily "I Didn't Raise My Boy to Be a Soldier" as the casualty lists from Europe became longer and longer. "Alexander's Ragtime Band" appeared in the same year as "I Want a Girl Just Like the Girl that Married Dear Old Dad" as the public still responded to the call of the settled past and tapped its feet to the rhythms of the new era. Henry Ford had pioneered the development of mass production manufacturing and the Model T's rolled off the assembly lines to the public's delight. Song writers celebrated the plight of the motorist-as-repairman with "Get Out

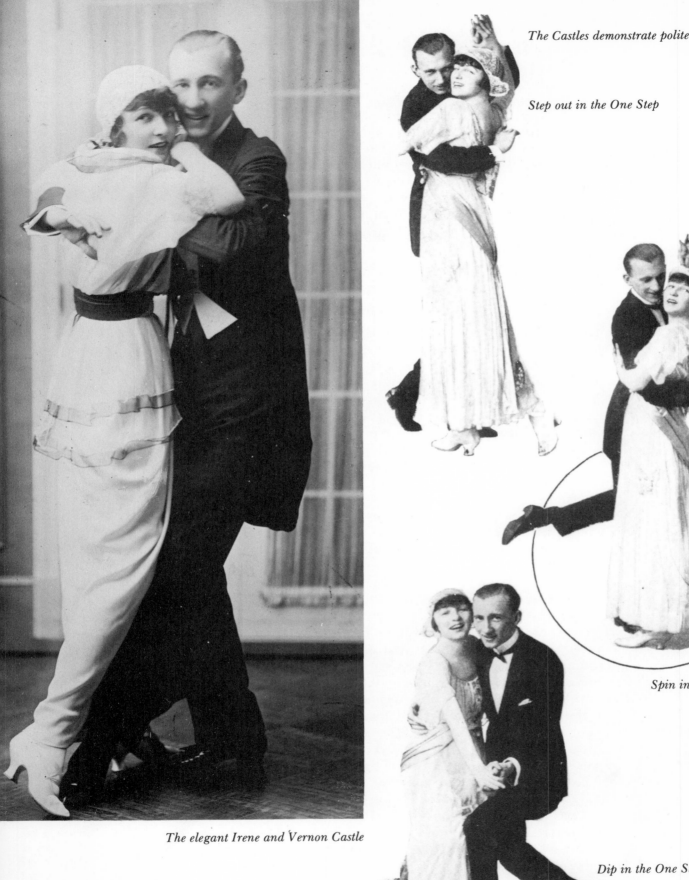

The elegant Irene and Vernon Castle

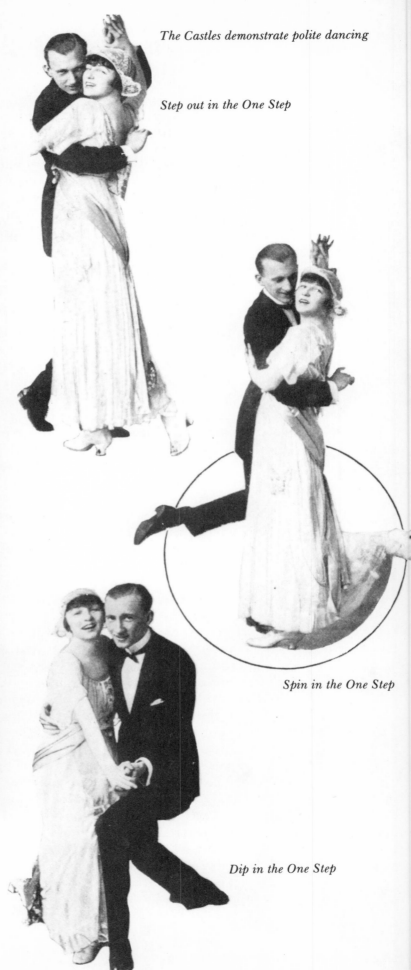

The Castles demonstrate polite dancing

Step out in the One Step

Spin in the One Step

Dip in the One Step

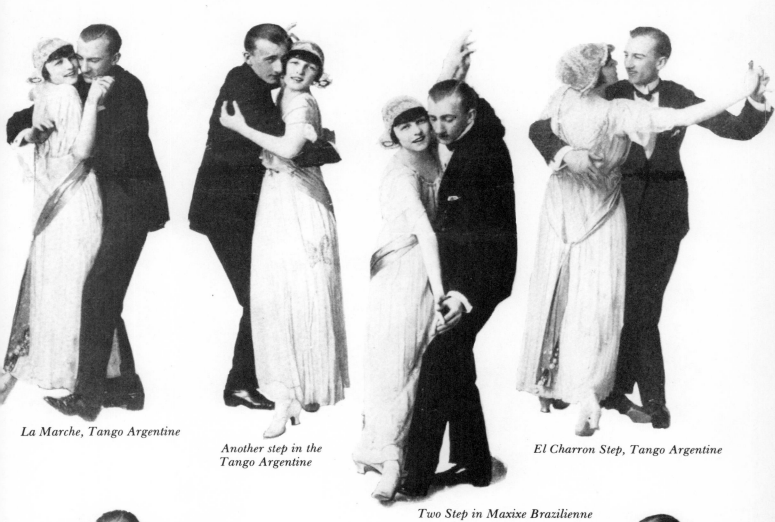

La Marche, Tango Argentine

Another step in the
Tango Argentine

El Charron Step, Tango Argentine

Two Step in Maxixe Brazilienne

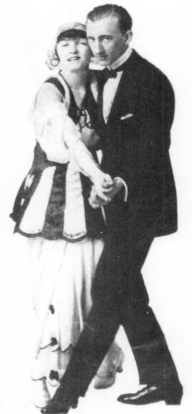

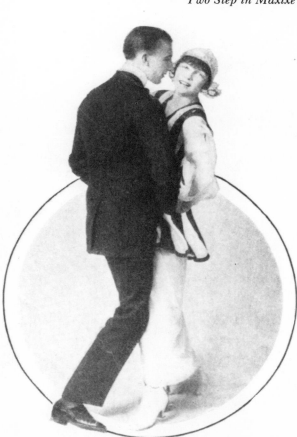

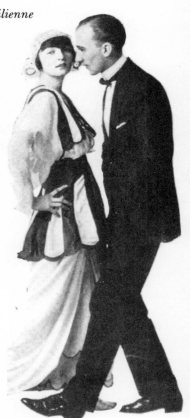

Promenade step in Tango Argentine

Media Luna, Innovation Tango

Corters of Innovation

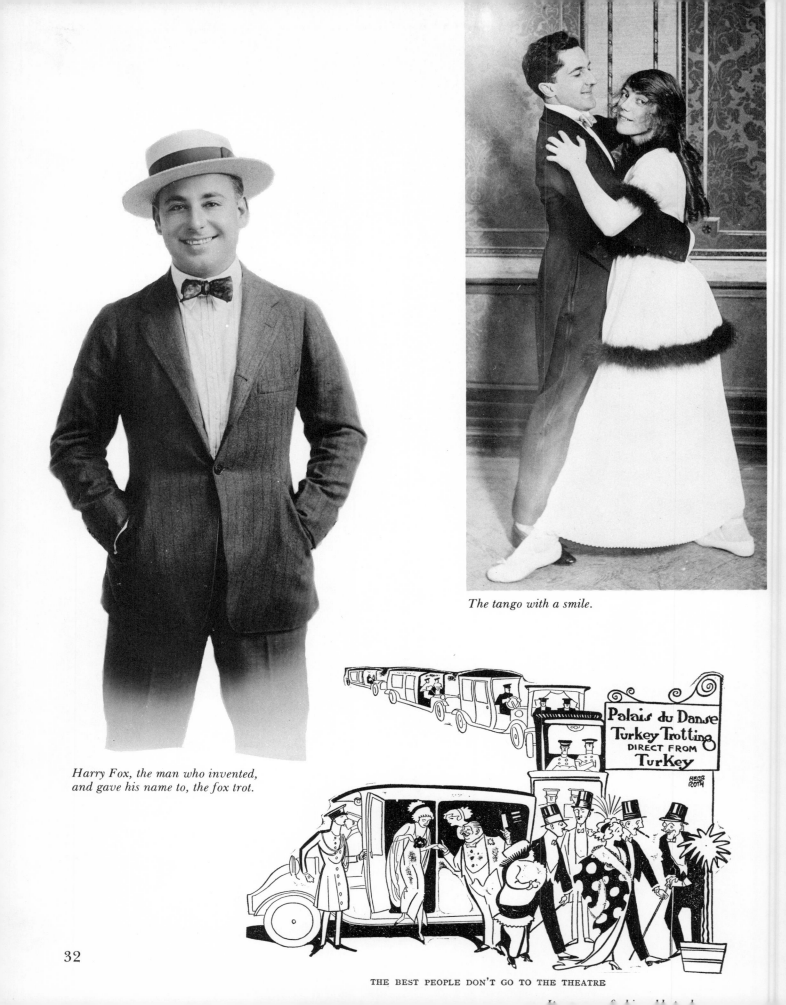

Harry Fox, the man who invented, and gave his name to, the fox trot.

The tango with a smile.

THE BEST PEOPLE DON'T GO TO THE THEATRE

Palais du Danse
Turkey Trotting
DIRECT FROM
Turkey

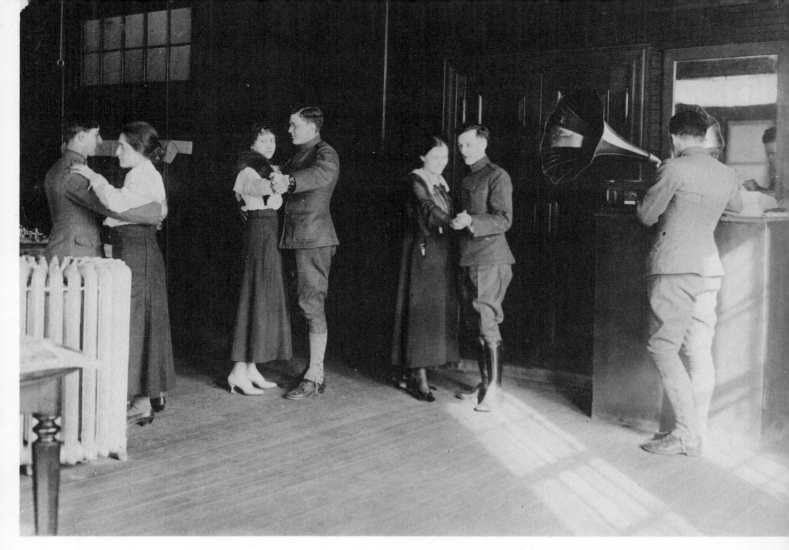

Soldiers and civilians dancing to Victrola music.

and Get Under" and black song writers were beginning to receive public recognition as William Christopher Handy ("Father Of The Blues") published the "St. Louis Blues" and Sheldon Brooks wrote the "Darktown Strutter's Ball." Social customs were changing in a variety of ways and the war accelerated most of the changes.

The portion of the decade that preceded the war was different in character from that which followed it. Despite its restlessness, it was much more innocent than the later years of the decade. The Castles could knock the rough edges off the menagerie dances before the war but one wonders whether they or anyone could have done much to tame the flirty, liberated dances that followed. Women started the decade with long hair and finished with it bobbed. Perhaps there had never been so shocking a physical change as when the new woman emerged without her "crowning glory."

The hem started to inch up almost as soon as the new decade began and ankles made an appearance. The size of hat brims began to diminish and become more sensible, and waists were fuller though they still remained

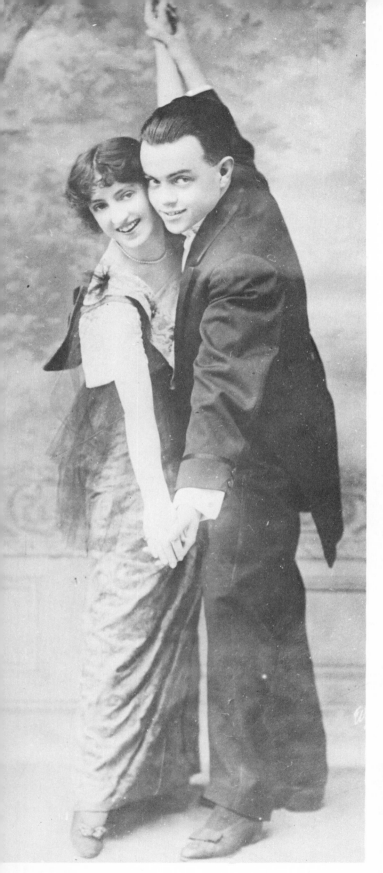

The maxixe, still unpronounceable but eminently danceable.

The maxixe which few could pronounce correctly but everybody did enthusiastically.

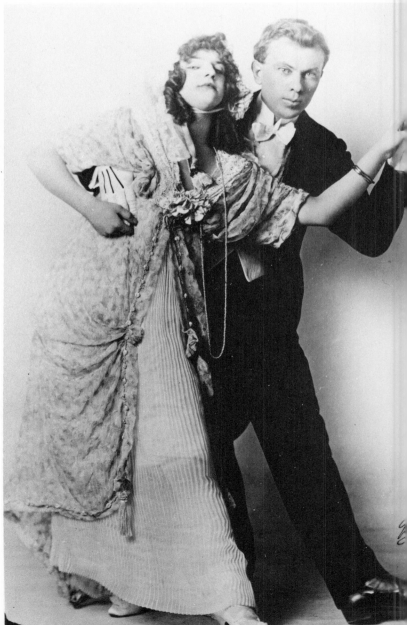

rather high. The tight-to-the-throat look, with severe collars, was banished in favor of a small V neck opening that was less constraining. Clothes were loosening up, perhaps a bit too much for some designers, because the hobble skirt suddenly appeared like a ball and chain intended to restrict women's movements. But it was a losing gambit and soon disappeared. Clothes were becoming more spontaneous looking and less laced-up. Bare arms were seen and in the evenings, a bit more décolletage was permissible. The fuller skirt moved right in after the hobble was banished and it became easier and easier for women to move freely.

Young women who wanted to make an independent point applied a touch more makeup to cheeks than society was willing to tolerate. Women were seen participating more and more in athletics and the war certainly hastened their appearance in a larger variety of jobs. However, women still could not vote and were arrested for protesting the ban in public places. Some aspects of the old ways held on. Even at the height of the dance craze, on the eve of war, *Ladies Home Journal* canceled a series of articles written

Side by side doing the tango.

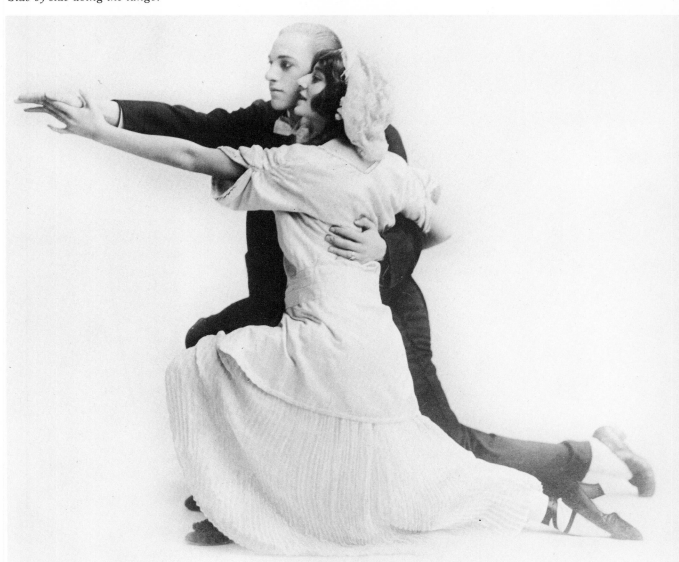

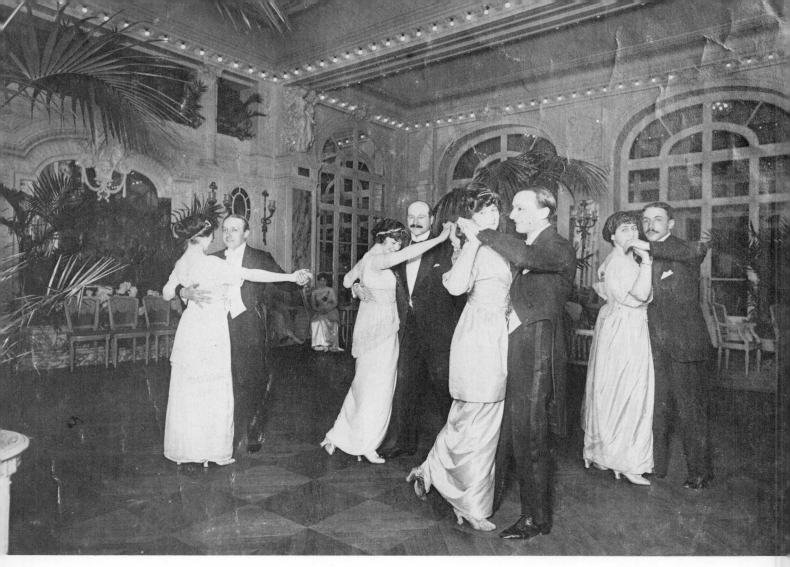

The dance floor, formal . . .

by the Castles to demonstrate the latest steps. Reader protest revealed an essential conservatism tht could still rear up when roused.

It's difficult to imagine what *Ladies Home Journal* readers saw that was objectionable in the dancing of the Castles, who were the last bulwark of the old sensibility. They danced closely but not inseparably tangled, and the Castle Walk was suavity itself. The couple walked forward, taking eight little steps and slightly rising up on the balls of their feet on the downbeat. Sometimes they would walk side by side for part of the pattern and then half turn, gracefully, toward one another before concluding it. While they moved around the floor a little zigzag pattern would appear as they crossed one foot in front or in back of the other; they could spiral down in ever diminishing circles and then just walk away. It was inspired walking and the public, the dancing public of the cities, loved both it and the Castles with their inventive, light, airy way of moving.

One critic said that Vernon Castle was the choreographic genius of the pair and that Irene was his finest creation. Irene didn't argue with the analysis and even included it among her reminiscences, *Castles in the Air*.

There were dozens of ballroom dance couples giving exhibitions, but none could compare in popularity with the Castles. Flocks of demonstrators sprang up in every city to perform in grills, cabarets, and ball-dining rooms, patterning themselves on the *thé dansant* model set by the Castles. The formula important for success was to have a lively couple to show the new twists and turns to the patrons who then swarmed onto the floor, virtually ignoring the food they had ordered in their rush to dance. Among the demonstrators, Maurice and Walton, Joan Sawyer and Jack Jarret, Mae Murray, Bonnie Glass, Irene Hammond and Arthur Murray were names that cropped up frequently as the public was seized by an obsession to dance. Before he started hearts fluttering from movie screens around the country, Rudolph Valentino danced with both Joan Sawyer and Bonnie Glass.

Dancers clasped one another cheek to cheek or walked along side by side. At times they moved in parallel patterns but avoided touching. They weren't compelled to face one another constantly but felt no hesitation about connecting closely when that was needed. Like the new loosening in women's clothing, there was a new spontaneity in the way that men and women danced. The war accelerated the velocity of social change.

There were still popular operetta composers like Emmerich Kalman, Rudolph Friml, and Sigmund Romberg who wrote the "Sweetheart" waltz

. . . and not so formal.

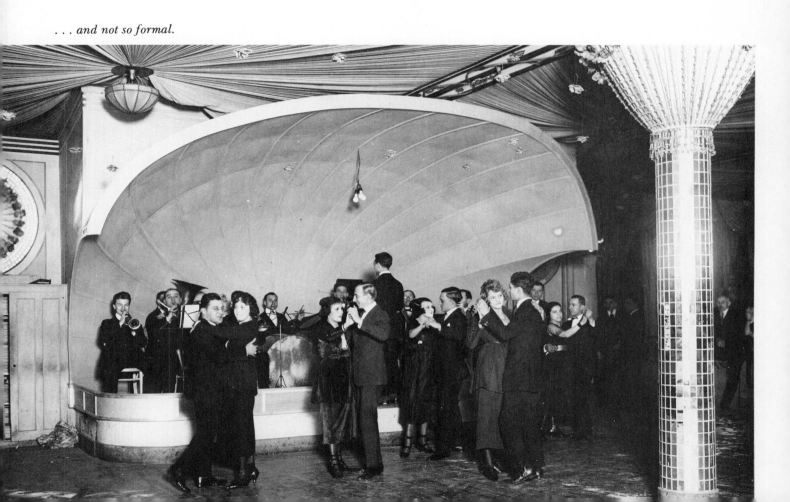

for his *Maytime* but there were significant new contributions from Jerome Kern, "They Didn't Believe Me" and "Till the Clouds Roll By." The prodigious career of Irving Berlin was moving into high gear as well, with "A Pretty Girl Is Like a Melody," in addition to his "Alexander's Ragtime Band" and his contribution to the war effort, "Oh How I Hate to Get Up in the Morning." George M. Cohan pitched in with "Over There." Congress gave him a medal and President Wilson sent along an autographed picture.

Florenz Ziegfeld was busy celebrating the American girl through his "Follies" which were extravagant costume parades set in the midst of

A smart evening on the town.

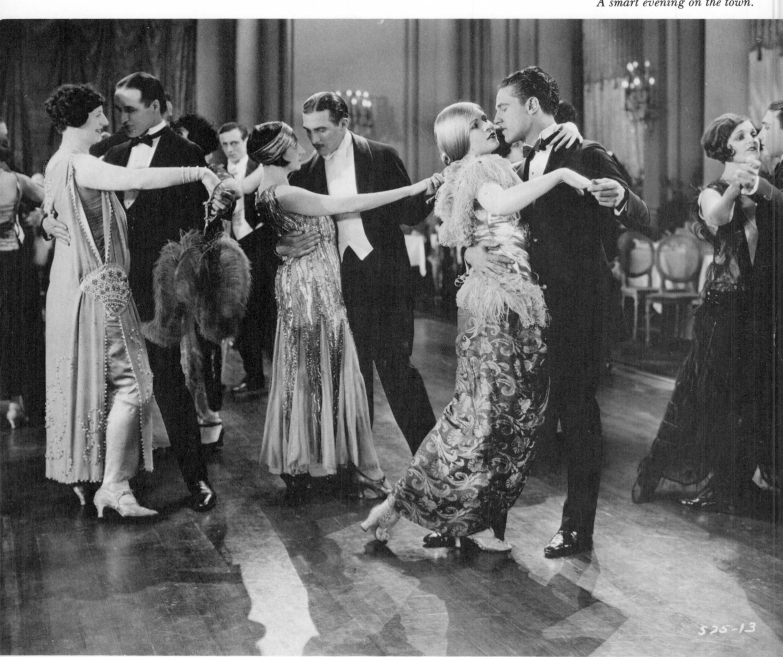

comedy sketches, songs, and parodies of Shakespeare, and a new sound was developing: jazz! It could be heard in the rippling bass line of the popular song "Dardanella" but was only beginning to poke its head up into the white culture from the world of black musicians who created it.

With one constitutional amendment, women were finally granted the right to vote and with another, everyone's right to drink was revoked. Composer Ernest J. Seitz wrote "The World Is Waiting for the Sunrise" for which future character actor Gene Lockhart fashioned the hopeful lyrics. Universal suffrage, Prohibition, and a hoped-for sunrise combined with bobbed hair, higher hems, and jazz to point the way to the twenties.

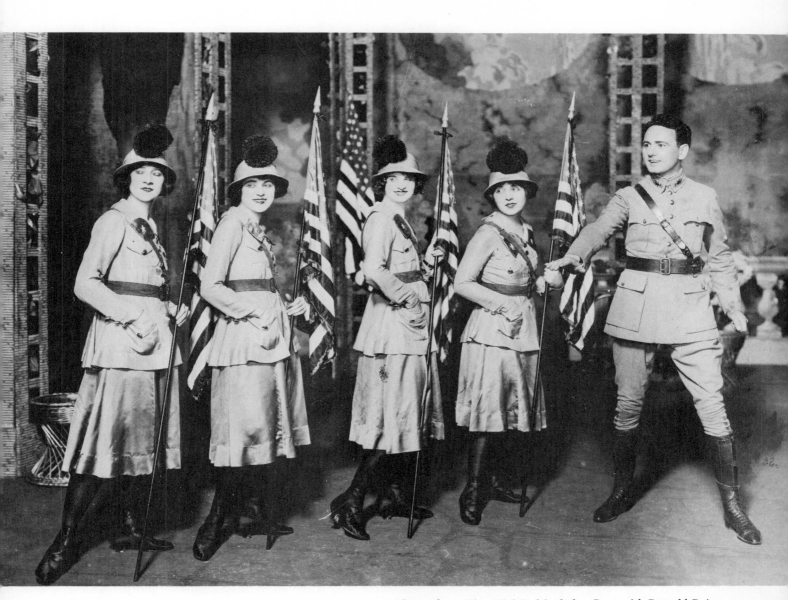

Scene from The Girl Behind the Gun *with Donald Brian.*

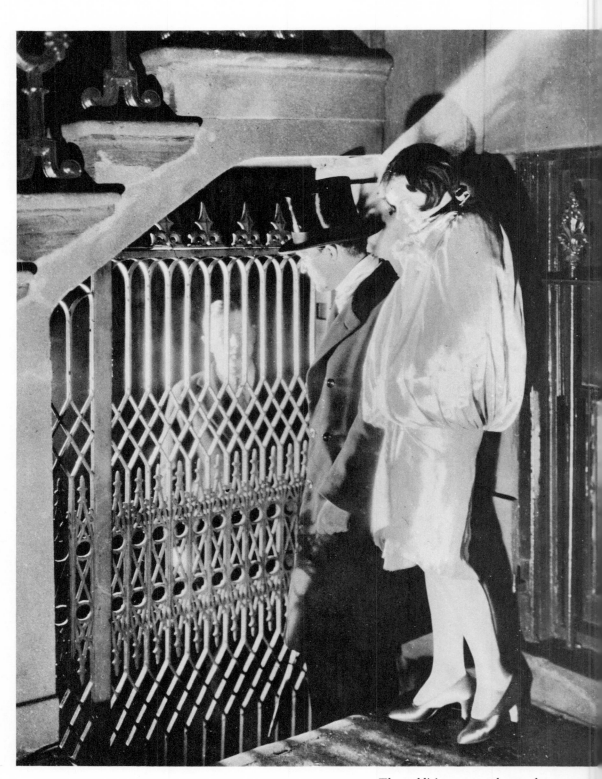

The public's answer: the speakeasy.

1920-1929

The nation celebrated prosperity and the end of
a successful war by thumbing its nose at the busybody "drys,"
who imposed Prohibition, and giving itself over to a succession
of fads. The boyish looking "flapper" carried a flask
of bootleg spirits in her garter, used "kissproof" lipstick,
and smoked as well. She also did the Charleston. But
the bubble burst when panic hit Wall Street.

JAZZ

In the weeks prior to January 16, 1920 when the Volstead Act officially took effect, the country prepared for Prohibition by buying and storing virtually every bottle of spirits it could get its hands on. No one knew quite what to expect, but everyone wanted to be ready. America was on the threshold of a golden age in sports, arts, entertainment, finance, exploration, and fads. George Herman ("Babe") Ruth would hit sixty home runs in a single season in 1927, an unheard of performance. Rosa Ponselle dominated the repertory of the Metropolitan Opera. Charles Lindbergh would fly the Atlantic singlehandedly. Admiral Byrd explored the Antarctic. Radio networks proliferated, men set records for sitting on flagpoles, marathon dancing appeared, and the first Miss America was crowned in Atlantic City. The stock market soared; prosperity had arrived with a rush. The war years were over and the country was ready for a celebration, but a willful majority of states insisted that it be a dry celebration. That made

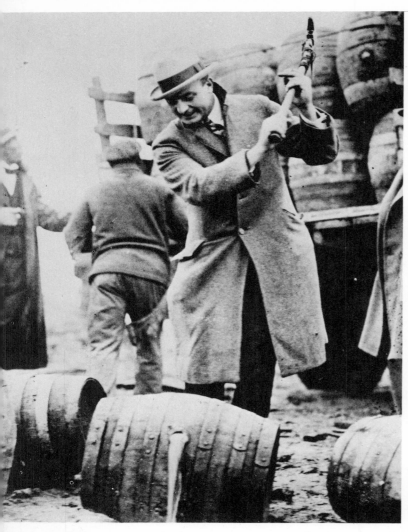

Prohibition.

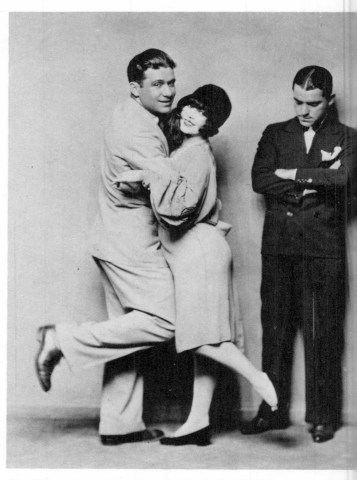

Tom Patricola and Ann Pennington do the Black Bottom under the watchful eye of George White, creator of The Scandals

little sense to the general populace, and organized crime flowered. Gangsters unexpectedly achieved a certain legitimacy by supplying what everyone wanted, much to the consternation of the holier-than-thou "drys."

The prewar days seemed remarkably remote to the young woman in bobbed short hair with her hemline at the knee and her dress waist dropped to circle the hips. She drew a bell-shaped hat (a cloche) down to just above her eyebrows and discarded the whalebone corset that had done so much to emphasize the upper torso look of the earlier period. The soft brassiere was introduced and many women suppressed any suggestion of a bosomy figure by binding themselves to appear flat. The streamlined look was in.

Women were beginning to function in what had been a man's world and they wanted to look their part. The smart young woman favored a boxy torso with de-emphasized bosom and hips, rammed a hat that looked like a helmet firmly on her head, had a mannish haircut, and strode about on newly liberated legs, of which a good deal could be seen. Jazz music abounded at the parties and entertainment spots that she frequented, and,

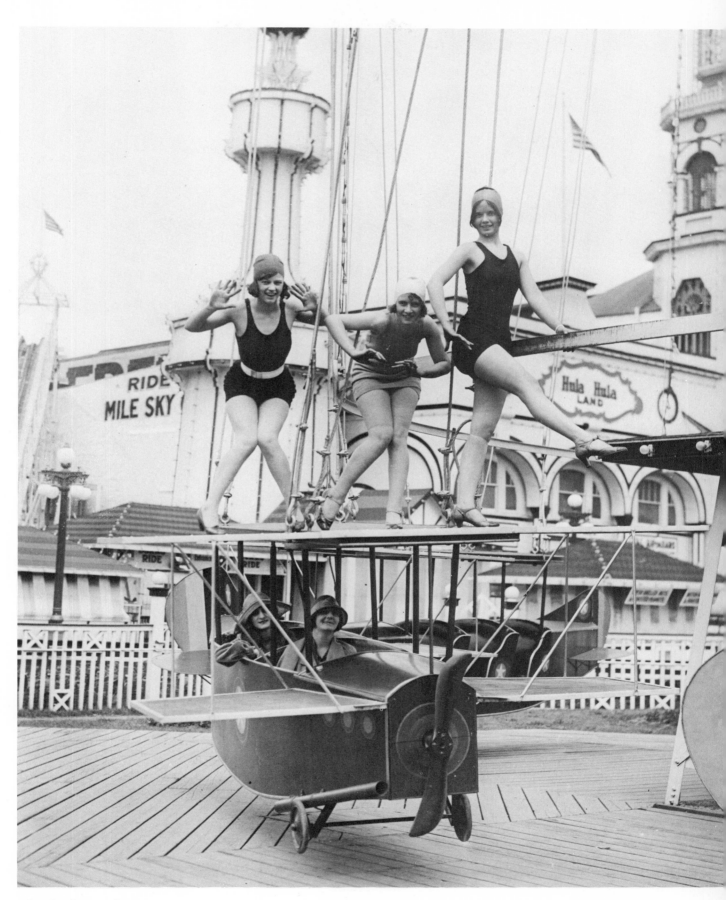

The Charleston, of course.

above all, she learned to dance the Charleston, flicking her knees open and closed with peekaboo insouciance. The pulpits roared their protest and averred that civilization, as it had been known, would never be the same. The young people had gone too far this time and before anyone could do a thing about it, they were dancing the Black Bottom, the Shimmy, and the Varsity Drag. Whew!

The *thé dansant* continued to be highly popular but it wasn't tea that was in the cups the revelers were drinking from. Hollywood introduced the talking picture with *The Jazz Singer* and a bevies of new singing and dancing stars flooded the screen. The archetypal flapper was Lucille LeSueur, born again on stage as Joan Crawford with her wide shoulders and energetic dancing which was seen in *Our Dancing Daughters.* Rudolph Valentino started as a male dancing partner in ballrooms and knew his way around the dance floor without any coaching. He might not have been a great horseman but he certainly knew how to tango. He popularized the sheik image of the daring loner pursuing a willing sheba who only made a pro forma objection to being swept away, and the strains of "The Sheik of Araby" poured from bandstands, radio loudspeakers, and phonographs.

The record business was booming with flat heavy discs that whirled wildly around at seventy-eight revolutions per minute delivering the sound individuals wanted, whenever they wanted it. They wanted dance music for the most part: "Tea For Two," "Varsity Drag," "Thou Swell," "I Want to Be Happy," "Gimmie a Little Kiss Will Ya Huh?," "Fascinatin' Rhythm," "April Showers," "Yes Sir, That's My Baby," "Who," and Tin Pan Alley provided all that anyone could ask for.

It was an age of imaginative slang in which the French chemise was familiarly known as a "shimmy." At one performance, singer Gilda Gray, who restlessly twisted and slithered while she performed, was asked what she was doing. She glibly shot back, "Shaking my shimmy!" and launched a new dance, the Shimmy. Performed in a tasseled or fringed dress it looked like the height of abandon: everything appeared to be going in every direction at the same time, and it became Miss Gray's signature piece. Soon America was humming and moving to "I Wish I Could Shimmy Like My Sister Kate." The Shimmy was a fad dance in a faddish age that spawned flagpole sitting, goldfish swallowing contests, and marathon dancing.

Though black musicians had always influenced white music, there were few opportunities for blacks to present their own music directly to the white public or be credited for it. During the twenties, however, black performers began to make an appearance on Broadway and in 1923 a black review, *Runnin' Wild,* featured a song accompanied by the dance that became the unofficial anthem of the decade: the Charleston. It was a dance that mother couldn't have done in a hobbled skirt, not by a long chalk. It couldn't even be done in the flowing, looser, long skirts of the previous decade, but it could be done in a short dress that gave ample opportunity for women to kick their legs and flick their knees. The flappers loved the Charleston and so did their escorts. It was bouncy and high-spirited and couples rocked and pitched around the floor. At times they hugged closely and then, just as jauntily, faced one another and cross-kicked. The smothering, dependent embrace that characterized the menagerie dances was not to the flapper's taste. Her clothes allowed her to move and she did so freely, letting the rolled-down tops of her stockings appear and disappear beneath the hem of her dress. The flapper's clothes didn't emphasize the "lower back" or the "upper torso" but the limbs. She swung her arms and legs so they looked as though they might fly off at any minute. She was free of the more onerous restraints of clothing, and other restraints were easing as well.

Few people drank as much before Prohibition as they did during it. No doubt the fact that liquor was forbidden gave a sharper edge to many thirsts. Women took up drinking the way they took up the Charleston, they started smoking in significant numbers as well. The advertisements smoothly suggested "Reach For a Lucky Instead of a Sweet," or pictured a pretty girl sitting near a smoking man with the invitation to "Blow Some My Way." Cigarette sales doubled, and the band played "Yes Sir, That's My Baby." Cosmetic sales grew as disapproval of their use lessened, and since Maurice Levy had invented the metal container for lipsticks during the war, they were now readily portable and convenient.

The young woman of the decade could vote, smoke, drink, use cosmetics freely, and hold a greater variety of jobs. It was also considered quite acceptable for women to engage in competitive sports. After all, if one could survive the Charleston, how frail and delicate could one be? William ("Big Bill") Tilden stood head and shoulders above any other male tennis player and his counterpart was Helen Wills, who might have lacked a sense of humor but was devastatingly consistent on the court. Glenna Collett slammed a golf ball with the best of them and Gertrude Ederle smeared herself with insulating grease and became the first woman to swim the English Channel.

In Chicago, the "King of Jazz," Joe ("King") Oliver, had settled in after starting in New Orleans to become the most respected and innovative jazz musician of the day. It didn't hurt that he had "Baby" Dodds on drums and Louis Armstrong on trumpet. Oliver's reputation was made in black clubs, but increasingly the white world became directly aware of him. Indirectly, white musicians tailored black jazz rhythms for white audiences. Bessie Smith was the acknowledged "Empress of the Blues" and those who visited black nightclubs were able to hear the young Duke Ellington, and Wilber de Paris. Eubie Blake contributed the title song to the black review *Shuffle Along* which came down from Harlem in 1925 to run on Broadway.

While jazz was making its impact, Latin rhythms also began to make a place for themselves. Reflecting on the appeal of the tango, which had been banned, characteristically, in Boston, band leader Xavier Cugat explained, "The tango is a very slow, sinuous dance with a mysterious and masked bass rhythm music. Tango lyrics are always tragic and even the music seems to carry the despairing wailing note." He recounted one that

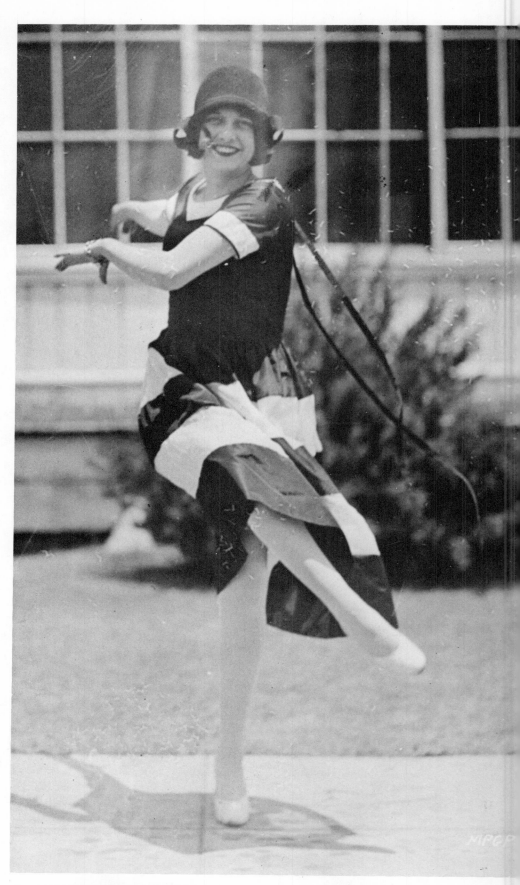

Joan Crawford and the Charleston.

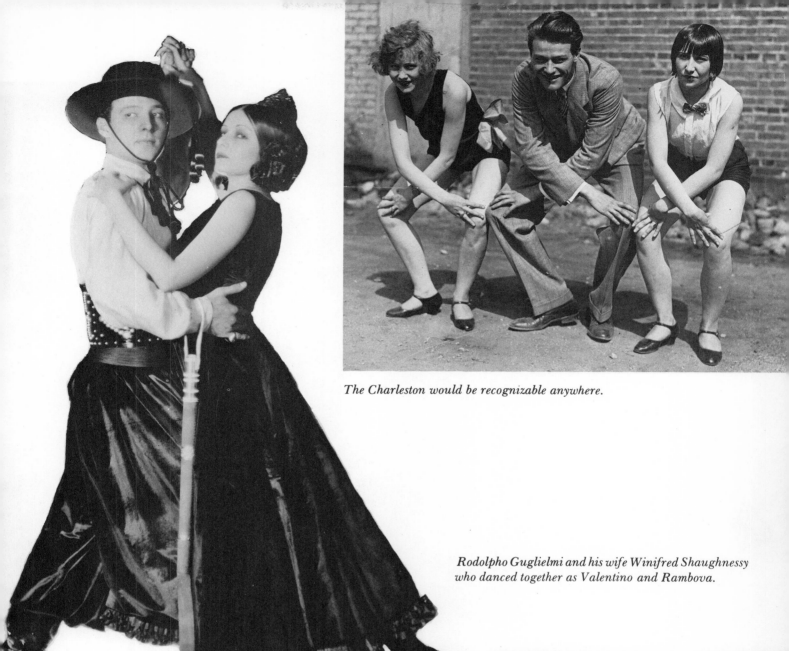

The Charleston would be recognizable anywhere.

Rodolpho Guglielmi and his wife Winifred Shaughnessy
who danced together as Valentino and Rambova.

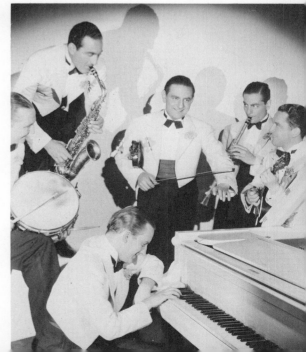

Guy Lombardo with "the sweetest music this side of heaven."

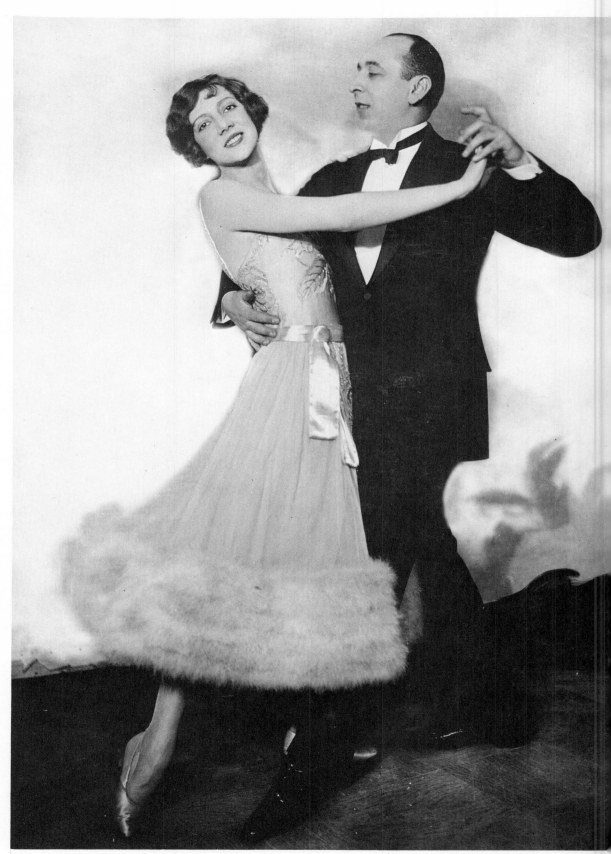

Arthur Murray in action . . .

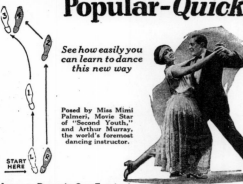
... and offering to teach anyone how.

"described almost every detail of how a boy finds his mother murdered and what his plans for revenge are on the murderer. The spirit of the tango is deep, sad, sentimental, languid, and at times quite morbid. The real tango is danced slowly and draggingly; the best dancers never lift their feet from the floor, but just seem to melt into each step, sliding their feet gracefully and beautifully. They appear to glide over the floor." The tango originated in the slums of Buenos Aires, surfaced in Paris and then came to the United States, but Americans found the rumba in Havana themselves.

Prohibition continued to be the national irritant. One tunesmith grumbled, "If I Meet the Guy Who Made This Country Dry." The cocktail, which was invented in America, couldn't be purchased there legally but enjoyed increasing popularity in Europe where it had recently been introduced. Fun seekers were attracted to the high life in Cuba and the songs noted "It Will Never Be Dry Down in Havana" or simply "I'll See You in C-U-B-A." While taking the local waters, dancers picked up a fondness for the lilting Latin rhythms and soon they were dancing them back home.

But alongside jazz and Latin rhythms there emerged a counterforce, the resurgence of an older, less hurried style of dance music. This was led by the gently phrased music of Guy Lombardo who moved into the Roosevelt Grill in New York and played 'the sweetest music this side of heaven' until his death, more than fifty years later. Lombardo displaced Ben Bernie, who was famous for saying "You Suh." George Eckhardt Jr., the director of the Hotel Mayfair orchestra, strongly disapproved of the boisterous music that was sweeping the land and stuck to a similarly conservative mode. He commented caustically, "With the Charleston came the blare of trumpet, the rasping notes of cornet and the pronounced clanging of cymbals. In other words the demand was for noise." Wayne King agreed and was dubbed "The Waltz King" in acknowledgement of his preference for three-quarter time.

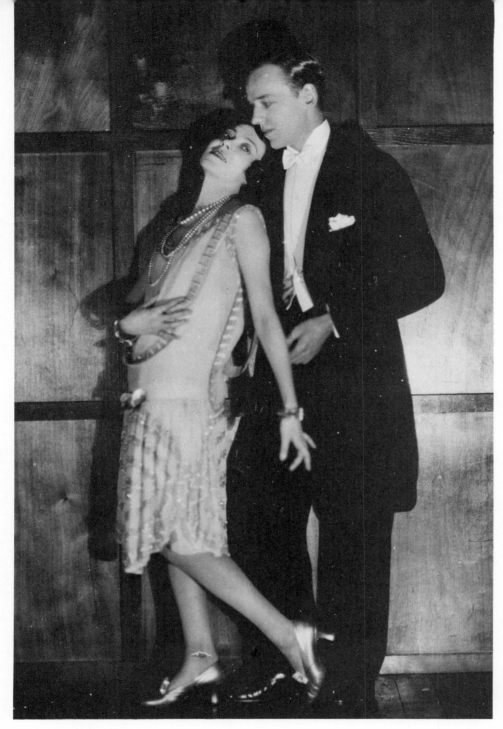

Adele and Fred Astaire.

Broadway was in its heyday with hundreds of shows, revues, follies, and vanities catering to the taste of an active theatergoing public. Audiences loved the Cansinos in John Murray Anderson's *Greenwich Village Follies* and later loved their daughter Marguerita who changed her name to Rita Hayworth and became a movie star. Grace and Paul Hartman, Maurice and Constance Talmadge, Ann Pennington, and a seemingly eternal Mae West, all made their mark, but a special niche was reserved for the Astaires, Adele and Fred.

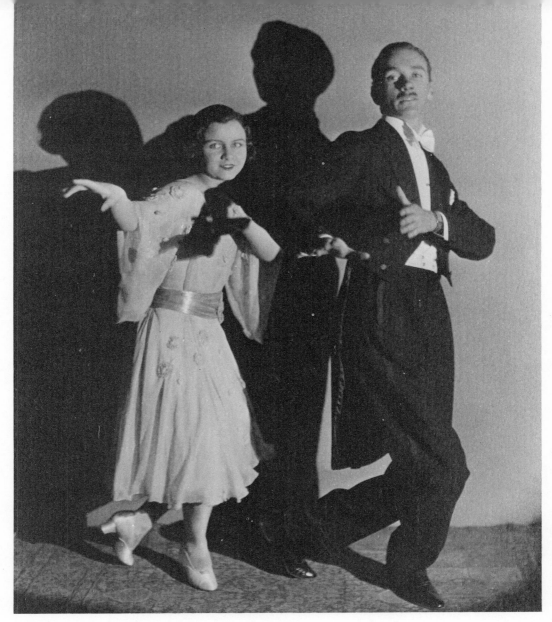

Mary Hay and Clifton Webb.

At the time, the public adored Adele and only really grew to appreciate Fred when he started to make movies in the thirties. They were an accomplished couple, with a special sense of comedy, and they graced the Broadway and London stage in a succession of shows during the twenties and early thirties. Adele married a titled Englishman, retired in 1932, and broke up the act. The brother and sister had gone about as far as they could go. They charmed the stage but couldn't dominate it romantically the way the Castles had. Fred had to wait for Ginger Rogers before that could happen. Since perfectly synchronized talking pictures were still a new medium and Fred understood their potential better than any other popular performer, that dominance was just a matter of time.

Webb Parmalee Hollenbeck was born in Indianapolis, but brought up in New York where his talent was spotted while in dancing school. However, he had to change his name to Clifton Webb before making his career on stage. He broke into show business doing demonstration dancing with Bonnie Glass, and later appeared with Mae Murray. He danced in Paris with Jenny Dolly of the Dolly Sisters and by the end of the decade had a striking success with a snake-hips solo he did while Libby Holman sung her way to stardom with "Moanin' Low." After switching to straight acting for the next thirty years, Webb plucked out a memory from his past during the fifties, by demonstrating a real Charleston to astonished undergraduates in *Mr. Belvedere Goes to College*.

The twenties went roaring on until the last quarter of its last year when everyone suddenly woke up to find that the stock market bubble had burst and the spree was over. They still danced, but there was a sour aftertaste. Revivalists Billy Sunday and Aimee Semple McPherson had preached hell-fire up and down the nation and it seemed on the point of realization. Even gang wars had taken on a particularly ugly tone with the multiple murders of the St. Valentine's Day Massacre. Far too many people had died or been sickened by impure bootleg spirits. The craziness of an era that embraced "Yes, We Have No Bananas" was ending and no one quite knew what was going to replace it. Hoagy Carmichael closed out the year by writing the lonely and haunting "Stardust."

"At last, at last, perfectly synchronized talking picture

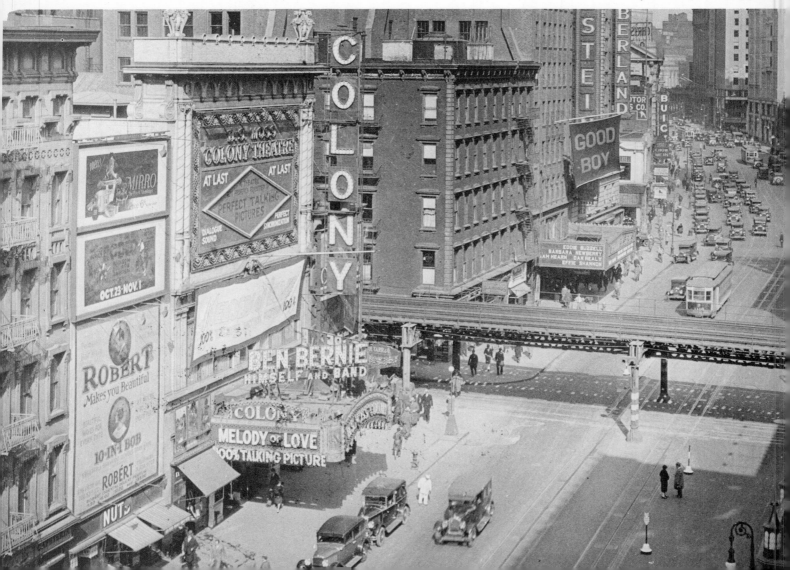

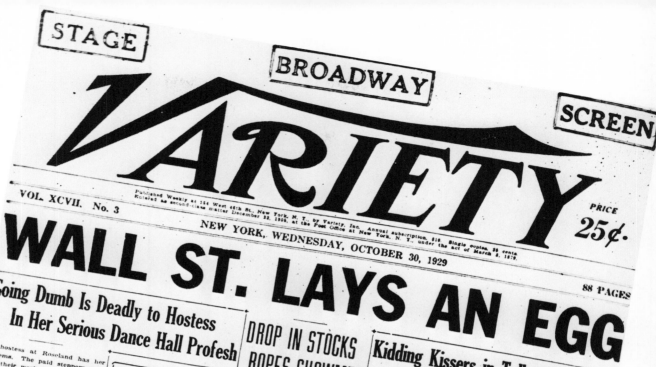

STAGE

BROADWAY

SCREEN

VARIETY

VOL. XCVII. No. 3

Published Weekly at 154 West 46th St., New York, N. Y., by Variety, Inc. Annual subscription, $10. Single copies, 25 cents
Entered as second-class matter December 22, 1905, at the Post Office at New York, N. Y., under the act of March 3, 1879.

NEW YORK, WEDNESDAY, OCTOBER 30, 1929

PRICE 25¢.

88 PAGES

WALL ST. LAYS AN EGG

Going Dumb Is Deadly to Hostess In Her Serious Dance Hall Profesh

A hostess at Roseland has her problems. The paid steppers consider their work a definite profession calling for specialized technique and high-power' salesmanship.

"You see, you gotta sell your personality," said one. "Each one of us girls has our own clientele to cater to. It's just like selling dresses in a store—you have to know what to sell each particular customer.

"Some want to dance, some want to kid, some want to get soupy, and others are just 'misunderstood husbands.'"

Girls applying for hostess jobs at Roseland must be 21 or older. They must work five nights a week. They are strictly on their own, no salary going with the job and the house collecting 10 cents on every 35 cent ticket. To keep her job, a girl must turn in at least 100 tickets a week during the cold season and 50 in the summer months. In a dull week girls buy their own tickets to keep up the record.

If a partner wishes to sit out a dance, he must pay for the privilege. "Sitting-out time" sells at eight tickets an hour, or $2.80. It's usually a poor sport who will come across with less than $2 many kicking in heavier for a little genial conversation.

The girl who knows her professional dancing trade will keep an alert eye open for potential "sitter-outers," ascertain their hobbies and talk herself into a whole string of tickets. In this way she not only earns money easily, but saves wear and tear on her evening dresses and slippers.

Big money rolls in if she has a good line. One of the most successful girls at Roseland takes this part of her work so seriously that she reads up on current events (sports and stock market included) and has a smattering of current literature and art.

"There are two types of hostesses at Roseland," she said, displaying high brow leanings. "They are the 'mental' and the 'physical.' Surprisingly enough the physical ones are not those who make the most money. One customer will buy three tickets from them at the most. They rely on their sex appeal and go dumb between dances—and that's the surest way to lose a partner, going dumb.

Mental Girls

The 'mental' girls, being good conversationalists, can wise-crack with the flippant, sympathize with the lonely and know how to salt the fresh boys and make them like it. I have one client who has been coming up every Monday night for two and a half years. Some times we dance all evening, other times we sit out every dance and just talk. He's a good spender, but his wife doesn't understand him."

Family the hostesses change every two years, although one or two girls have been there for eight years. Some marry, some go into show business, others get hot checking for chorus, others are

Hunk on Winchell

When the Walter Winchells moved into 204 West 55th street, late last week, June, that's Mrs. Winchell, selected a special room as Walter's exclusive sleep den for his late hour nights. She shushed the Winchell kidlets when her husband dove in at his usual eight o'clock the first morning.

At noon, Walter's midnight, his sound proof room was penetrated by so many high C's he awoke with but four hours of dreams and a grouch. Investigated at once, after having signed the lease of corse.

Right next door, on the same floor, is the studio of the noted vocal instructor, Kinney. Among his pupils are Ona Munson, Irene Delroy and Marjorie Peterson. They love Winchell like you love carbolic acid.

And Miss Munson is reported to have requested that an amplifier be started hereafter when she runs up the scale.

Demand for Vaude

Springfield, Ill., Oct. 29.

Petitions requesting Publix theatres to resume vaudeville in Decatur, Ill. are in circulation in that city.

Petitions specify that vaudeville at one or more of the three larger Publix houses would furnish employment to a number of Decatur musicians and stage hands and provide larger variety of local entertainment.

Paul Witte, Publix manager in Decatur, states that he believes vaudeville will find a place in Decatur before the season is over.

Pickpocketing Dying Out

Chicago, Oct. 29.

Some 1,000-odd pickpockets who used to make Chicago what it was are no more. A confidential list in the hands of government revenue men shows them to be operating in bottles.

In the last eight months there has not been a complaint or an arrest for pocket picking.

Flirting Contest

Paris, Oct. 29.

New idea here, a flirting contest at the bal Tabarin. Contestants are permitted to flirt only to a limited degree with a committee of judges regulating their manner.

DROP IN STOCKS ROPES SHOWMEN

Many Weep and Call Off Christmas Orders — Legit Shows Hit

MERGERS HALTED

The most dramatic event in the financial history of America is the collapse of the New York Stock Market. The stage was Wall Street, but the onlookers covered the country. Estimates are that 22,000,000 people were in the market at the time.

Tragedy, despair and ruination spell the story of countless thousands of marginal stock traders. Perhaps Manhattan was worst hit in the number of victims. Many may remain broke for the rest of their lives, because the money that disappeared via the ticker tape was the savings of years.

Many people of Broadway are known to have been wiped out. Reports of some in show business losing as much as $300,000 are hearsay. One caustic comment is that was that the theatre is enough of a gamble without its people to venture into Wall street.

Prominent showmen, several identified with the picture industry (Continued on page 64)

FILTHY SHOW OF SHUBERTS GOOD FOR SCREEN

Chicago, Oct. 29.

Shubert's latest musical of their "Night" series, now in Chicago, is so filthy that one of the cast admits embarrassment while in the performance.

The second act of this scramble called "Broadway Nights," is the (Continued on page 63)

Soft Drink Smuggling

Chicago, Oct. 29.

Bootlegging, charged water and ginger ale into the main Loop hotels is recent.

Water, at hotel prices, is 45 cents a bottle. Under the new plan a bigger bringe in a case at 25 cents a bottle. Ginger ale coming through three channels retails at 18 cents. Hotels get 50 the bottle.

Kidding Kissers in Talkers Burns Up Fans of Screen's Best Lovers

Talker Crashes Olympus

Paris, Oct. 29.

Fox "Follies" and the Fox Movietone newsreel are running this week in Athens, Greece, the first sound pictures heard in the birthplace of world culture, and in all Greece, for that matter.

Several weeks ago, Variety's Cairo correspondent cabled that a cinema had been wired in Alexandria, Cleopatra's home town. Only Sodom and Gomorrah remain to be heard from.

HOMELY WOMEN SCARCE; CAN'T EARN OVER $25

No homely ones on Broadway! And now it looks as if Crosby Gaige may have to postpone production of "One Beautiful Evening" because the Main Stem is devoid of the non-beauts necessary for the casting of the show.

Arthur Lubin, caster for the producer, for several weeks has been trying to land the right type of women. A most unusual piece, the drama has an all-women lineup, and, although as many as 22 are needed, all must be homely—and middle age or over, except for two who can be young.

Vera Caspary wrote the play and it centers about conditions at a club for girls where requirements of residence demand that the girls must not earn over $25 per week in order to live under its roof. That's why they must be homely.

Ads for Execs

Chicago, Oct. 29.

Newspaper ad calling for potential executives for the Publix-B. & K. organization here, drew heavy response, with over 100 applicants. From all walks of life, with several $20,000-a-year men among the mob, seeking a chance to break into the show business.

Studio in Church

A new Roman Catholic Church, Holy Angels, newly opened on East 47th street near 1st avenue, New York (Italian Parish), has rented out its upper story as a motion picture studio.

Vitagraph, industrial picture concern, has established its head-

Boys who used to whistle and girls who used to giggle when love scenes were flashed on the screen are in action again. A couple of years ago they began to take the love stuff seriously and decided but the talkers are reviving the ha ha for film osculators.

Heavy loving lovers of silent picture days accustomed to charm ing audiences into spasms of silent ecstasy when kissing the leading lady are getting the bird instead of the heartbeat. The sound accompaniment is making it tough.

Such a picture romancer as John Gilbert is getting laughs in spite of the sighs of other days, and the flaps who still think he's grand are getting sore. One little flap had is quieted by an usher when making a commotion during a Gilbert picture at the Capitol, New York. The person sitting next to her, like many others in the house, too, jumped to his defense and started to bawl out the Gilbert derider.

Not only has Gilbert received the bird lately, but all of the other male screen players who specialize in romance, Charley Farrell in "Sunny Side Up" draws many a giggle from his mush stuff.

In the silents when a lover would whisper like a ventriloquist, his eyes apart and unmoved, and roll to the clinch and then kiss, it looked pretty natural and was believable. The build-up to the kissing now makes a gag of the kiss. When the kiss is on with section intent, the laughs are out of order. It's burning the impressed female fans to see their favorite kissers kidded when kissing.

In Reverse

Seems the only type of love stuff received as intended since advent of the talkers in the comedy love scene. The screen comics are becoming the heavy lovers and the heavy lovers comedians.

The normal kiss, delivered with the usual smack, sounds like an explosion. For that reason talkers had them rolling in the aisles.

Toning down their kissing to make it noiseless has made bum kissers of the screen's best lovers, but, audible or silent, the kisses are getting laughs that don't belong.

Hollywood, Oct. 29.

Soft- pedal on dialog in romantic love scenes in the future. Here-after, the saccharine stuff will be (Continued on page 63)

BROOKS COSTUMES

Big business panned by show business.

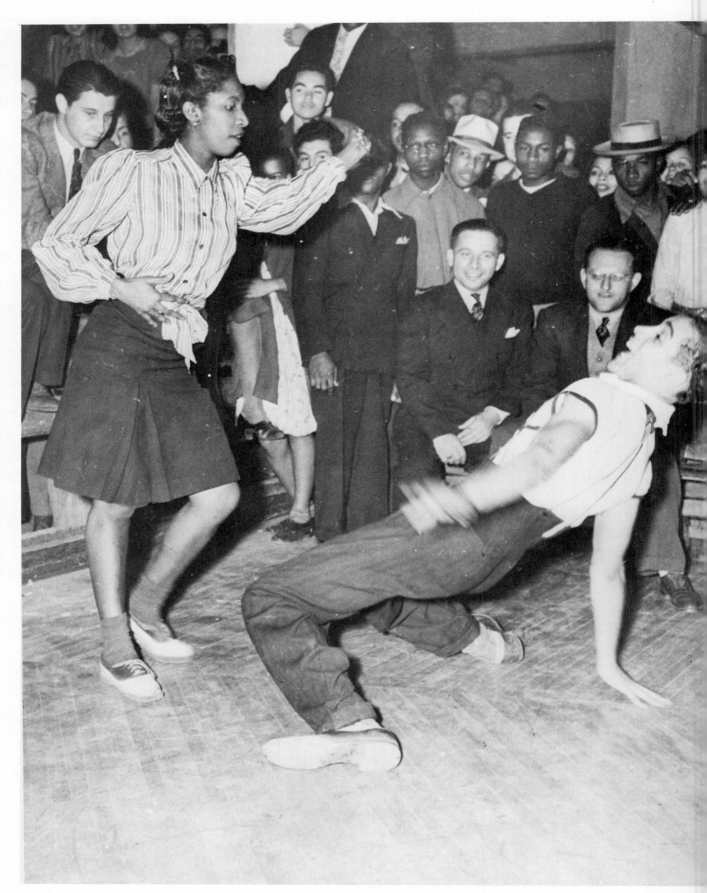

Jitterbugging on the ground . . .

It was the era of the big bands in which lively jazz dancing took people's minds off the great Depression, and marathon dances awarded prizes to the survivors. While no one could easily forget hard times, better times were on the way and the country hosted two world's fairs in anticipation of the world of tomorrow.

SWINGTIME AND MARATHONS

The grimness spread slowly but eventually a third of the country was unemployed and the majority barely getting along. Day-to-day life was difficult and became increasingly expensive as incomes shrank.

Clubs declined, and after 1933, when the Volstead Act finally was repealed, the speakeasies disappeared. It became much more economical to entertain at home and when people threw a party, it might just be a rent party to pay that month's lodging. The rise of the radio networks played a big part in providing the music that accompanied such parties and the popular figure was the young couple "cutting a rug," i.e., dancing at home in the living room, or the parlor, as it was less and less often referred to.

There still were lots of dance bands but the kids most frequently gathered at one another's homes or at the ice cream parlor where the jukebox would unfurl yards of danceable music for five cents a play. The dances were increasingly influenced by the jazz arrangements known as

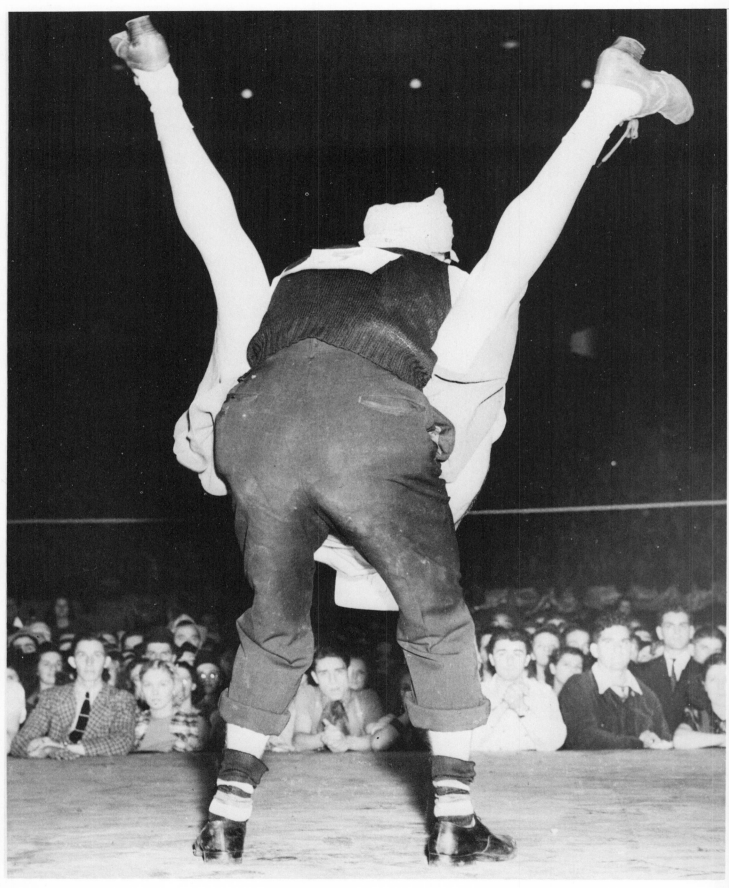

. . . and in the air.

swing. Swing dancing was even more athletic than the Charleston and the dancers were getting younger and younger. Adults still covered the dance floors in the clubs but the neighborhoods were dominated by the kids and before the decade was out they would be dancing in theater aisles to the sound of the "King of Swing," Benny Goodman.

The big dance was the Lindy-Hop which originated in Harlem's Savoy Ballroom as a dance rendition of Charles Lindbergh's (Lindy's) big hop across the Atlantic in 1927. The freedom which had been developed with the flying arms and legs of the Charleston, Black Bottom, and Varsity Drag now took on an airborne aspect that began to look like acrobatics when the best dancers did it. The boy and girl stood face to face in an athletic stance in which feet were braced apart, knees flexed, and crooked fingers firmly locked together to form a good coupling. The woman was tossed into a blizzard of turns and supported jumps that did indeed look like indoor flying.

With her right hand firmly hooked into his left and the other lightly draped on his right shoulder, she placed her weight on the balls of her feet, raising her heels slightly. His right hand was touching her waist as they stepped to the syncopated beat that shifted rhythmic emphasis from the normal to the unanticipated counts. A light push from him would send her in a half turn out and away and she would return on the next count. If the push were inward she did a full circle under his raised arm and close in the familiar starting position. A few torso twists in unison and they were ready for the next "flight" which could be a double turn. The combinations were almost infinite for the really imaginative and the "double" was a variant on the full inward turn. After she had completed the rotation and was again facing her partner, he bent smoothly toward her, placing her right hand behind her back and grasping it with his right while pulling her toward him. When the Lindy was properly executed the young woman looked like a top with her hair flairing out. The considerate partner avoided vertigo by varying the directions of the spins and occasionally tossing in a two-hander. The partners stood face to face grasping hands, then simultaneously twisted inward while raising high one pair of hands and rotating under them while releasing the other. Skirts were creeping higher and higher, so that for competition couples underwear was as important as the skirt itself.

In the movies, almost everybody danced, none more stylishly than Fred Astaire with Ginger Rogers. They were the best that the decade had to offer and, in their way, as dominant as the Castles had been, even though many dancing teachers complained that they did not interest themselves sufficiently in the ballroom dance scene to offer the real leadership they were capable of. But something had happened that was not amenable to any type of imposed leadership. For the most part people were not coming to dance teachers for instruction in the mainstream dances, but were asking for the latest fad dance which the schools themselves had not really had a chance to analyze and assimilate. It was a chaotic time, since dances

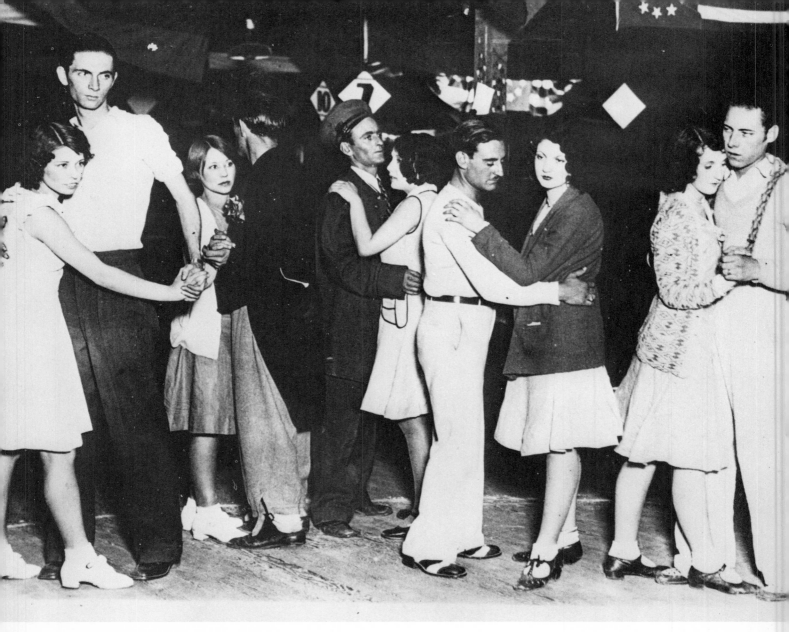

A dance marathon, and the strain shows.

appeared and disappeared with eye-dazzling rapidity and the teachers felt themselves a bit lost without a set repertoire of approved dances to teach. Since everybody danced, they did the best they could. In Boston, of course, the "recognized" dance teachers banned cheek to cheek dancing, "not on the grounds of morals but on the ground of awkwardness." Tell it to the Marines!

In Europe people were upset because of the spontaneity of the new American dancing. They wanted to have fixed patterns, not anarchy. American social dancing looked haphazard from across the water but really was a strong expression of individuality. The best teachers devoted themselves to keeping track of the fads and trends and to preparing their pupils to move spontaneously and creatively themselves. One of the most alert and enterprising teachers was Arthur Murray who through his

Benny Goodman, the king of swing.

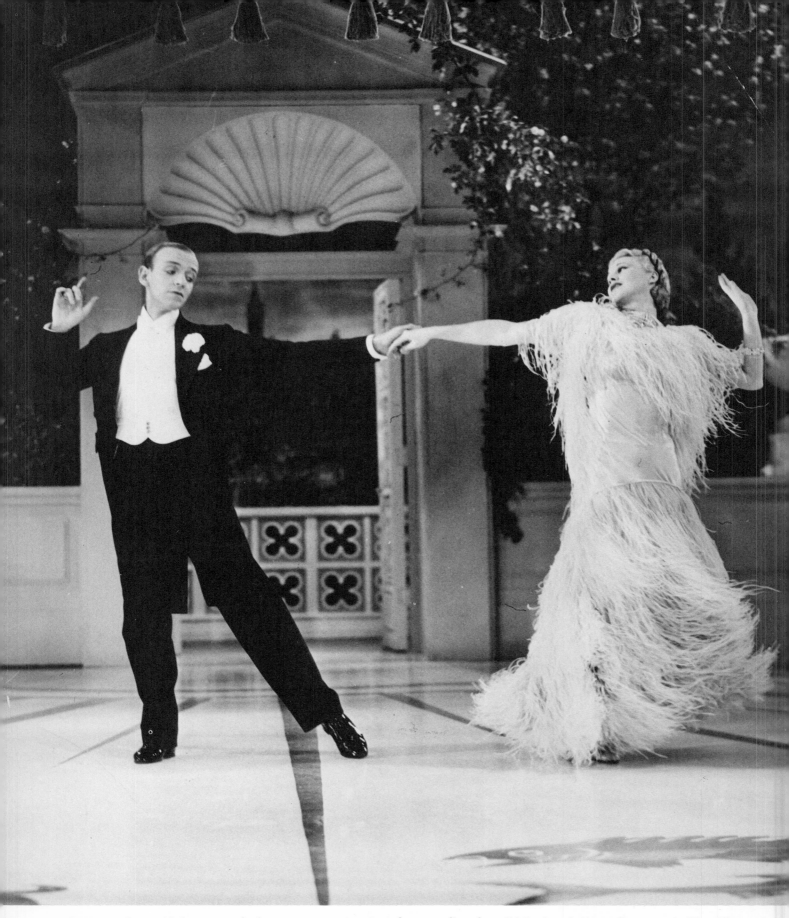

Dance teachers said that no one had ever sent more people to dance studios than did Fred and Ginger, here seen in Top Hat.

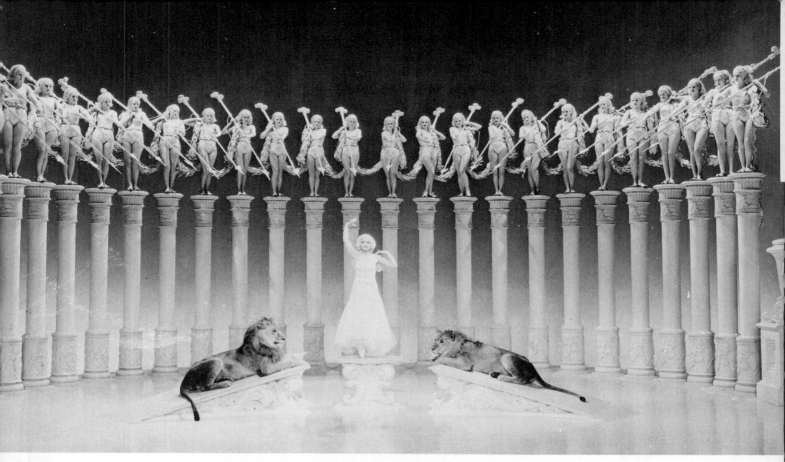

Florenz Ziegfeld loved spectacle so the movies provided plenty in The Great Ziegfeld.

studios and home instruction courses literally taught millions to dance. He operated with a combination of good business sense and a keen eye for the significant new dances. His greatest coup was his domestication of the Big Apple.

The dance was first noticed at a roadhouse in North Carolina called The Big Apple and Murray went down to see what was developing. What he saw was a country jazz dance that combined swing and square dancing, with a caller and all. By the time he was finished with the Big Apple, Murray had incorporated elements from a variety of dances, plucking out steps from the shag, Suzi Q, and Truckin' and blending them into the basic circle that provided the dancing space. The couples started in a parade and then joined hands in a large circle facing in toward the center.

The caller would indicate one or another couple who would move to the center to do an individual variation, to "shine" as in "Shine the Apple." Sometimes they "peeled" the apple and other times they "cut" it, but they always returned to the big circle and periodically rushed to the center waving their hands in the air to "praise Allah." "Truckin' " was done with a rise and sag of the shoulders while one partner waggled a fist overhead with the forefinger pointing straight up. The shag was a fast-hopping dance with a little kick in back and a stomping motion with the front foot. The Suzi Q characteristically had the fingers of both hands interlaced at chest height with the elbows straight out to the sides so that one could make a "sawing" motion across the body while doing cross-over steps. Elements of the Charleston and of the Black Bottom, with its hip slaps, crept into the Big Apple which accommodated them all with a slaphappy, egalitarian grace.

There was a grim side to social dancing which was expressed in the marathon contests. These were endurance events and no mistake. The last couple left standing won. The typical marathon held out a glittering grand prize to the couple who would endure the necessary agony; and in a time when jobs were scarce people were willing to try anything. Dance styling was never a part of marathons, only endurance. Dancing was variously interpreted but the basic requirement was that the couple kept moving, shuffling, dragging, anything so long as it was the soles of the feet and only the soles of the feet that touched the floor and the couple maintained some type of continuous motion. There were ten-minute breaks every hour and the participants snacked six times a day, that is six times in each twenty-four hours, and did their sleeping on the dance floor as they groggily moved around enough so as not to be eliminated. Hallucinations were frequent; dancers hardly knew where they were and would wake up with a start to find themselves locked in their partner's arms and just barely moving along. There were circuits of marathon dancers and hardened couples moved from one show to the next. The smart ones toughened their feet by dipping them alternately in hot and cold baths before the contest started. People participated because the dance marathon offered a chance to make some real money.

If everyday reality was grim, Hollywood definitely was not. The studios cranked up the dream machine full blast and in his heyday Busby Berkeley was using those dancing darlings Dick Powell and Ruby Keeler with a supporting cast of thousands. Berkeley provided spectacle and escape for a public that adored both. If one violinist was good, then a hundred would be great, reasoned Berkeley. If one twinkle-toed couple dancing up and down a flight of stairs was exciting, then fifty would be stupendous. So it went through all of his musicals. He multiplied the ordinary until it became extraordinary and then filmed it from angles that made it look even more exciting. The "Gold Diggers of 1933" hopefully sang "We're In The Money", and in 1935 the public was treated to "The Lullaby of Broadway."

It was the classic period of the musical. How could it be otherwise with George Gershwin, Jerome Kern, Irving Berlin, Cole Porter, and Arthur Schwartz all turning out shows on Broadway and in Hollywood? *Girl Crazy* introduced Ethel Merman singing "I Got Rhythm," "Gay Divorce" became "Gay Divorcee" as a movie, and Fred and Ginger looked ravishing dancing to the "Continental" and "Night and Day." They were so good that it almost wasn't fair. The movies not only made money but established a pattern of popular classic dancing that has not been surpassed. "Dancing in the Dark" emerged as the big hit from *The Band Wagon,* as "Begin the Beguine" and "Just One of Those Things" were from Porter's *Jubilee.* Everybody danced.

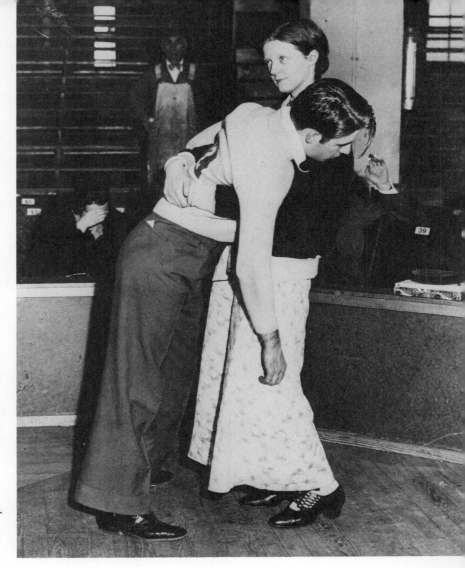

Even the spectators look exhausted.

James Cagney started out tap dancing and ended up shoving a grapefruit into Mae Clark's face in *Public Enemy*. Buddy Ebsen danced until they turned him into a hillbilly and George Raft aspired to artistic fulfillment in *Bolero* until it was decided that he made a much better box office attraction as a tough guy. Shirley Temple tugged at the nation's heartstrings and Bill ("Bojangles") Robinson dazzled them with his tap artistry. They were too good a pair for the studios to mess up and so they were left alone. Clifton Webb had been invited to Hollywood to make musicals but before the studio was finished with him, he was playing a psychopathic murderer, John Philip Sousa, and a bullying babysitter. *O tempora, O mores!*

Women decided to appear womanly again after the boyish look of the twenties. The helmet was replaced by hats with broader brims and the sculptured flowing style was favored in dresses. It was a little severe, especially with the hemlines dropped down so that the knees vanished, but the times were stressful and frivolity seemed inappropriate in day-to-day things. The face became a mask of contrast with eyebrows pruned to a thin arched line and lips fully shaped and dark to bring out the pallor of the

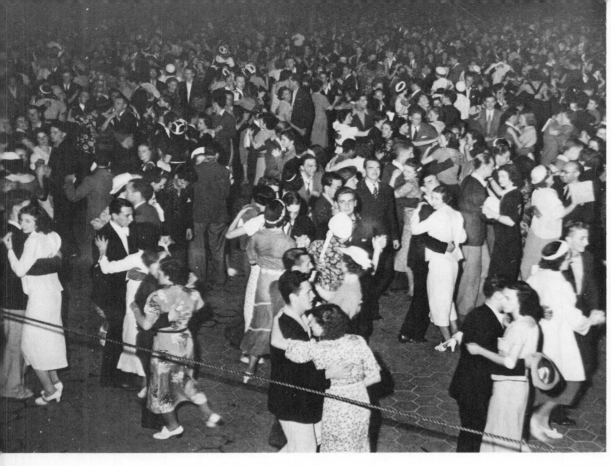

Dancing in New York's Central Park . . .

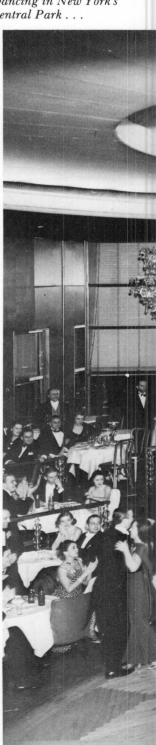

skin. Makeup was an acknowledged part of every woman's armament and she didn't wait until age thirty to start using it, as Harriet Hubbard Ayer had suggested she should before the turn of the century. Waves began to appear in the hair, which was still kept short. The art deco look dominated buildings, interiors, and faces.

Inexpensive entertainment in the form of radios and movies absorbed leisure hours and the family radio was one of the most substantial pieces of furniture in the living room. People looked at it as they listened to the messages that were broadcast and it seemed as if the person speaking was in the room with them. The messages came in contrasting forms. Franklin Delano Roosevelt delivered reassuring "fireside chats" to the nation, encouraging good sense in difficult times, while the fiery and fabulously successful radio priest Father Charles Coughlin sounded a stridently intolerant note in political discourse. Millions heard the ringside commentary as Joe Louis took the world heavyweight title from James Braddock and reacted with horror at the news broadcasts that told of the war clouds spreading over Europe again. Things were tough enough without another war.

The lack of cash drove some men and women to the simple expedient of bank robbing. There was a Wild West air of romanticism about the robbers' dash-and-grab style of life. At least they were doing something about the pressure that everyone was feeling. But the law didn't see it that way; before the decade was out John Dillinger, Bonnie Parker, Clyde Barrow, and Pretty Boy Floyd were all gunned down by the forces of law and order

64

while other gangsters were packed off to prison. The worst of them ended up in Alcatraz, the newly created maximum detention prison in San Francisco Bay, grimly known as "The Rock."

Saturday night was the big date night and the radio stations transmitted hours of music for party-goers to roll up the rug and dance. Programming began in early evening and carried on until late at night as station after

. . . and overlooking the park in the "Rainbow Room."

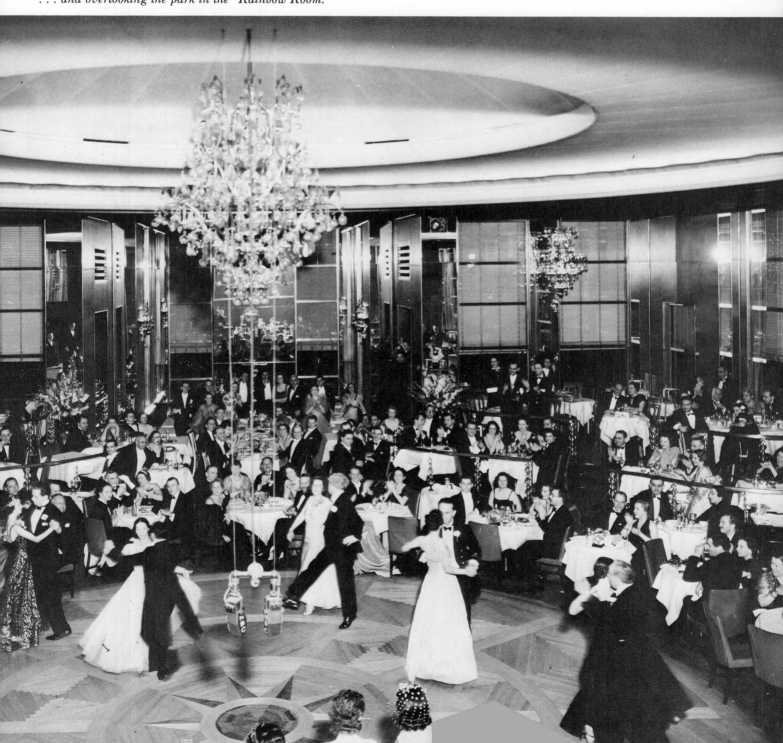

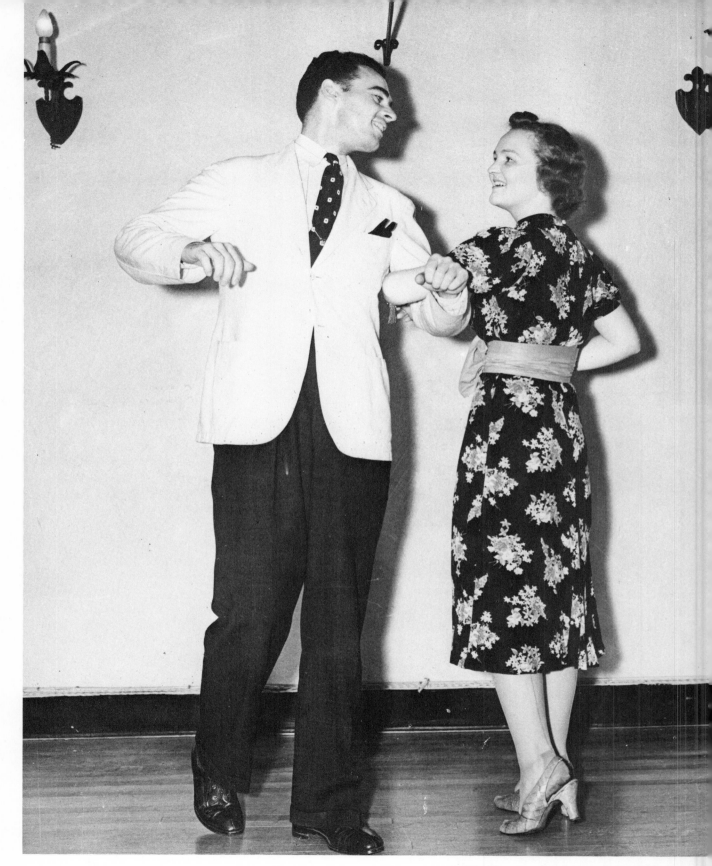

Hooking arms in the Lambeth Walk . . .

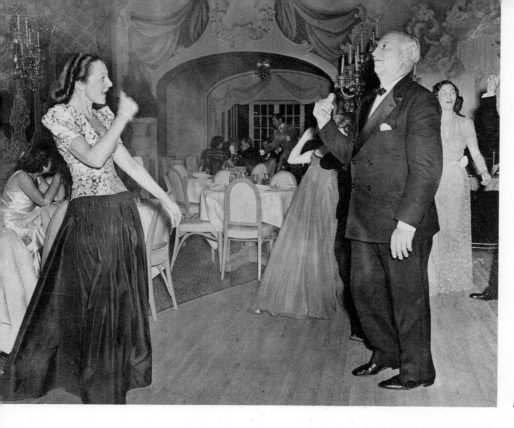

*. . . and tossing a fist over
the shoulder while saying "Oy!"*

station joined the network from the various time zones across the country.
The big bands were those of Benny Goodman, Glenn Miller, Artie Shaw,
Harry James, Tommy Dorsey, Duke Ellington, Count Basie, and Xavier
Cugat who supplied the Latin rhythms. Kate Smith sang "God Bless
America," Bing Crosby's signature tune "When the Blue of the Night
Meets the Gold of the Day" was heard, and the public indulged its fancy for
loony songs with the "Hut Sut Song."

By the close of the decade, things were on the upswing economically and
the country splurged on the New York World's Fair and the San Francisco
Fair simultaneously, both of which offered a glimpse of the world of
tomorrow. Television was first seen by the mass public, the Trylon and
Perisphere dominated the skyline in New York's Flushing Meadows Park,
and the giant red National Cash Register totaled the number of daily
visitors, in the window where the dollars and cents usually appeared. The
curious from all over the country, as well as from abroad, swarmed in. A
funny cockney dance, the Lambeth Walk, became a fad as couples slapped
their thighs, walked side by side, hooked one another's arms, then separated to toss a clenched fist over the right shoulder with an extended
thumb while saying "Oy!"

The Disney Studio's *Snow White* had a gaggle of songs that accurately
reflected the prevailing moods, with praise of work in "Heigh Ho" and
"Whistle While You Work," and hope for the future, in "Some Day My
Prince Will Come." People danced to "Deep Purple," "All the Things You
Are," "Embraceable You," "Dancing in the Dark," "September Song,"
"Anything Goes," and the rousing "Pennsylvania Polka." The darkest
economic days were past, and the country looked forward to a new era of
prosperity.

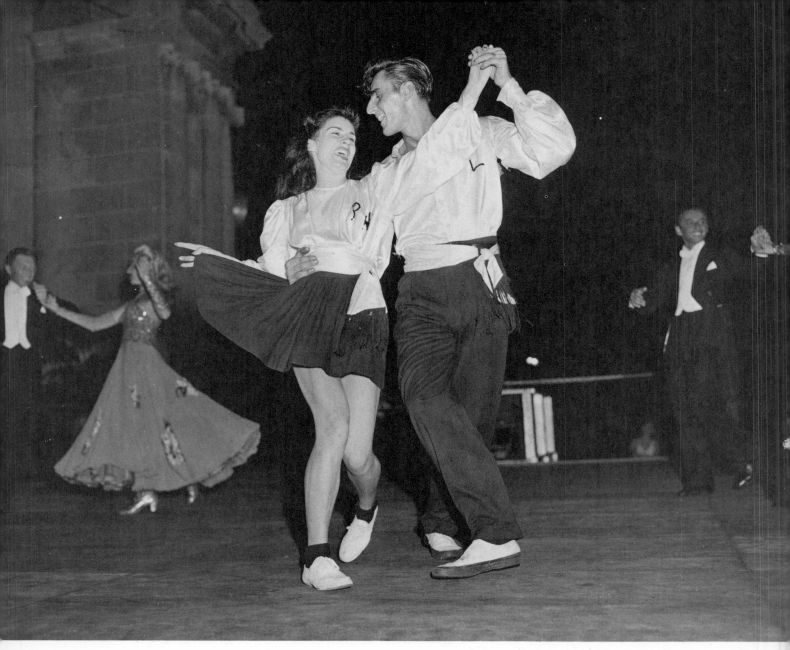

Competition couples. The ones in sneakers are jitterbuggers.

1940-1949

Jitterbugging and the samba were the big dances,
though World War II absorbed the country's energies
during the first half of the decade. Afterward,
everybody began to enjoy themselves again.

JITTERBUGGING

America's cherished business indicator, the gross national product, was up a whopping 10 percent over 1939, the country jauntily elected Roosevelt to an unprecendented third consecutive term, and the average age was sixty-four as opposed to forty-nine in 1900. Conditions close to home looked a lot better than they had in quite a while. Women's hemlines continued to rise and comedians made rude jokes about this on the airwaves and were reprimanded for doing so. Women's shoulders broadened to mannish width with the addition of padding, the well defined waist stayed in its natural place, and little hats clung to the tops of heads as women stepped along on platform shoes.

Technicolor movies were becoming more frequent on the screens that normally showed black and white films almost exclusively, and the development made it possible for women to match the exact shades of lip, eye, and finger coloration of their favorite stars. Max Factor, who designed

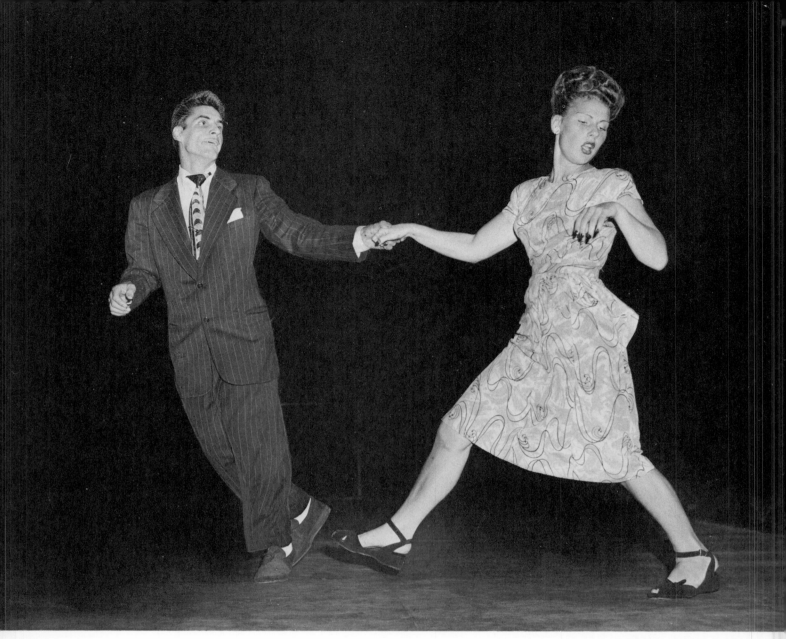

A guy and his girl struttin' their stuff.

"makeup for the stars" made his cosmetic line available to any woman who desired it. The Second World War, which began in Europe in 1939, made itself felt in America's life two years later, as did the "war face," designed by cosmetician Elizabeth Arden. It emphasized a determined, almost hard look that persisted through the decade, though modified somewhat after the actual shooting had stopped.

As men disappeared in increasing numbers into the various branches of military service, they were steadily replaced on the "home front" by women; the legendary figure of "Rosie the Riveter" emerged. She kept her long hairdo tied up inside a kerchief while working around machinery, wore coveralls, and pocketed a healthy paycheck for her labor. She was tough and independent, and when she went dancing, the jitterbug seemed like the only logical dance for her. It was rough-and-tumble, hectic, and reflected the times. Left to their own devices while husband or boyfriend

70

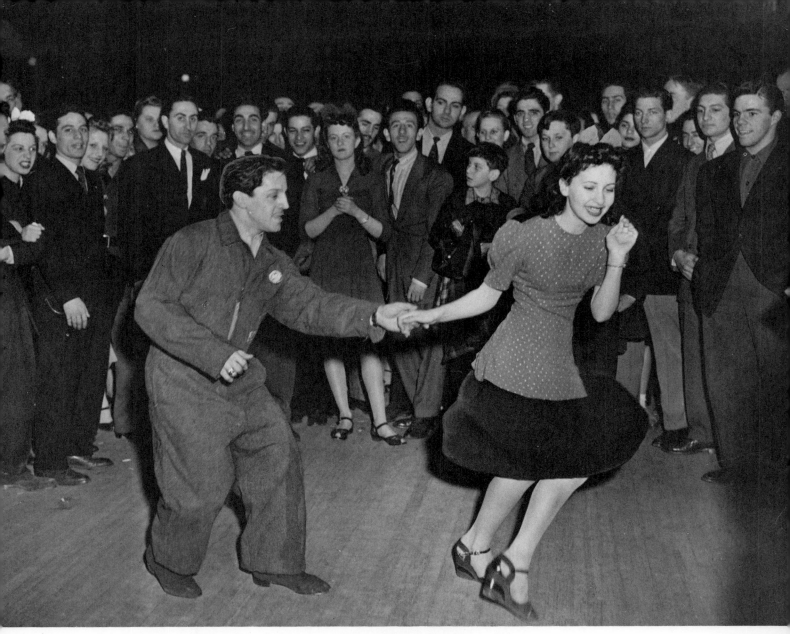

Defense workers get together for a Sunday afternoon dance away from the plant.

was away, women found that they could manage lots of jobs that they had never thought seriously of before. "Rosie" might have been a stereotype, but she expressed the determination to carry on, despite the shortages imposed by the war effort. Nylon stockings, which had only begun to appear toward the end of the thirties, were a conspicuous casualty when the armed services discovered myriad uses for the tough, lightweight, artificial fiber that came out of a nozzle. "Rosie" darned and made do; in extreme emergencies, she painted her legs.

The generation that had grown up in the thirties was a hardy breed and turned a tough exterior to the world that was expressed in flip chat with a rapid-fire delivery. "Jeet?" translated into "Did you eat?" and a typical boy-girl dialogue might run like this: He: "You dancin'?"; she: "You askin'?"; he: "I'm askin'!"; she: "I'm dancin'!" When things were going well, musicians and civilians thought that everything was copacetic.

Fashions were being pushed to extremes by both men and women. At the outer limits, gentlemen's jackets were padded to the point of no return. Some looked as if the hangers had been left inside when they were donned and the baggy trouser leg was "pegged" to an ankle-hugging tightness. In some cases the normal opening was too small to accommodate the foot and the trousers were zippered at the ankles to permit the wearer to slip them on and off. It was the time of the "zoot suit" which required a "reet pleat" for full effect. An oversized snap-brim fedora was *de rigueur* as well as a large curving key chain that was attached to a belt loop and plunged to the knee or lower before nestling in the gentleman's pocket. Thus attired, he sought out his girl on the ballroom floor.

Her jacket was padded in the shoulder as was his and her hem stopped at the knee or above. Her dancing shoes were likely to be two-tone saddle shoes with the lace-up "saddle" and heel panel in brown leather and the rest white. If she wore a sweater instead of a jacket it was big and bulky and she favored thick, white, athletic, "bobby" socks—hence the term bobbysoxer. When the spirit moved her, she slipped into the aisles of big movie theaters which had live attractions as well as movies and she danced.

Social arbiters decried this behavior aloud and frequently feared for the future of the country if these were to be the mothers of the next generation. The future mothers were having too much fun to pay attention. They were also discovering a thin, young singer with a big baritone voice who sang first with the Harry James orchestra and then went to Tommy Dorsey's. He heralded the end of the docile band singer who sat on the sidelines, for the most part, while the big bands played, then approached the microphone on cue to render a number and return to his place on the bandstand.

It soon became apparent that the young women were much more interested in Frank Sinatra's voice than they were in the bands that had been the dominant attraction. When they heard that beautifully phrased voice croon it made them faint, or swoon as it was called, and "The Voice" was launched as an independent performer. The days of the big bands were numbered, although the decline stretched over a period of fifteen years.

In the meantime, the bands played on. When the musicians were inducted into the service, they played in military uniform. All the major cities set up recreation centers for servicemen who always seemed to be in transit from one place to another. On the West Coast, San Francisco was the big port of embarkation for the Pacific theater of operations and on the East Coast, it was New York from which men were directed into the European and North African campaigns. Broadway put its best foot forward by creating the biggest, most glamorous, entertainment center under the guidance of the United Service Organizations and called it the Stage Door Canteen. A popular song related how one young man left his heart at the Stage Door Canteen and one of the dancing standouts at the servicemen's balls was "Killer" Joe Piro. He was untiring and seemed capable of dancing all night with a variety of partners; he became a star in his own right. It made people feel good to see such energy and verve.

Uptown in Harlem, it was particularly lively at the Savoy Ballroom on Tuesday nights when the "Four Hundred" Club gathered to dance. These were the avid, and most skilled, devotees of jitterbugging; membership in this "Four Hundred" was dependent on ability and enthusiasm. A jitterbug was a slang term for a fast dancing partner and it soon came to describe the sort of dancing that they did as well. The bounce that was inherent in the Lindy was developed into gymnastic aerial moves that sent young women flying perilously toward the ceiling from whence they would swoop down to be caught and held momentarily before being launched again. The couples developed fierce rivalries and the dancing became wilder and wilder as they tried to outdo one another. It was frantic, athletic as a sporting contest, and ferociously exhilarating.

On Broadway there was a little dance revolution of its own developing and the most prominent example was *Oklahoma!* The choreographer Agnes de Mille had created a "dream" sequence in dance movement that was not merely an interlude but an integral part of the story and advanced the plot. For the next decade and a half, dream sequences were an essential part of the Broadway musical. The first musical with a scoundrel for a hero, *Pal Joey,* appeared and focused public attention on the formidable talents of Gene Kelly.

In 1940 the New York World's Fair, which had opened in 1939, closed its gates but many of the novelties introduced during its run stayed on to become regular parts of peoples' lives. Papaya juice enjoyed a new vogue in North America and so did the samba. As part of its contribution to the Fair, Brazil had built a national pavilion and had sent along a samba orchestra to play the lilting, flirtatious rhythm to visitors. It was the time of the "Good Neighbor" policy when the United States government began to treat South American nations as partners in the Americas, rather than as awkward geographical accidents. The State Department even sent American Ballet Caravan, precursor of New York City Ballet, on a South American cultural friendship tour.

There was an appeal to the samba which was based, in part, on its own merits and in part on its being a halfway house between the more conservative forms of social dancing and the exuberance of jitterbugging. The rumba had paved the way in the previous decade but despite its below-the-hips sinuousness, the upper body was still and it was danced mainly in a single spot. What was now needed was a dance that had an unusual and provocative rhythm but that traveled around a bit, though not excessively, and also gave some interpretive options to partners about the use of the upper body. It was almost as if the samba had been created to fill the void. Dancers who were still intrigued with fast dancing, though not prepared to cut loose completely, did like the energy expressed in the samba. Combined with the new interest in things south of the border, the samba was ushered into clubs and ballrooms with considerable success.

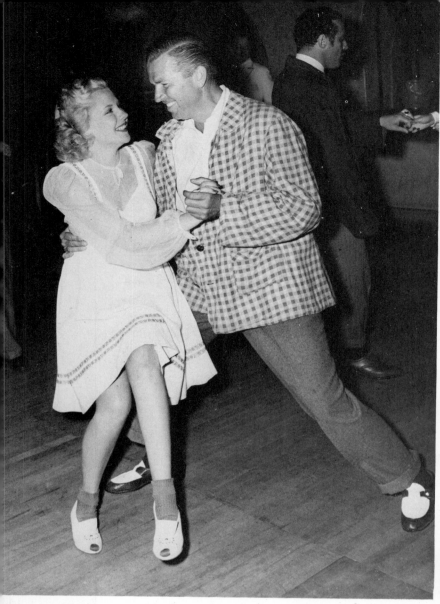

Movie stars Marie McDonald and Bruce Cabot at a "zoot suit" party.

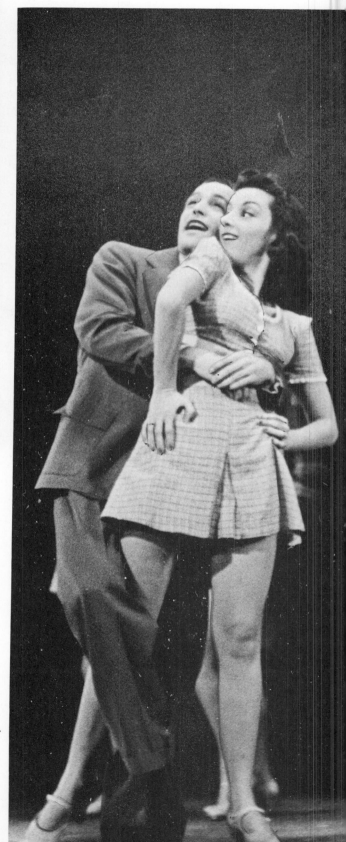

Pal Joey *and its rascally star Gene Kelly.*

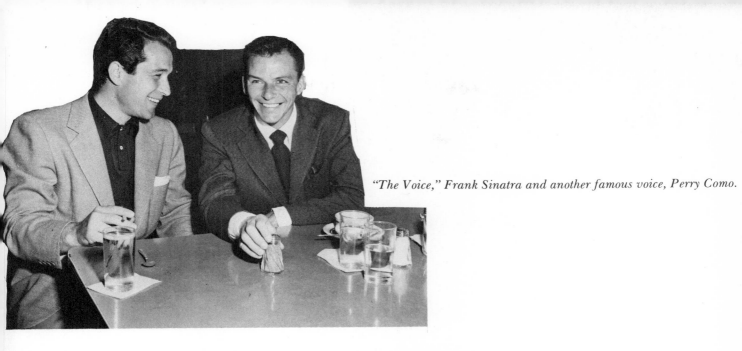

"The Voice," Frank Sinatra and another famous voice, Perry Como.

Rita Hayworth leads the conga line at the Stage Door Canteen.

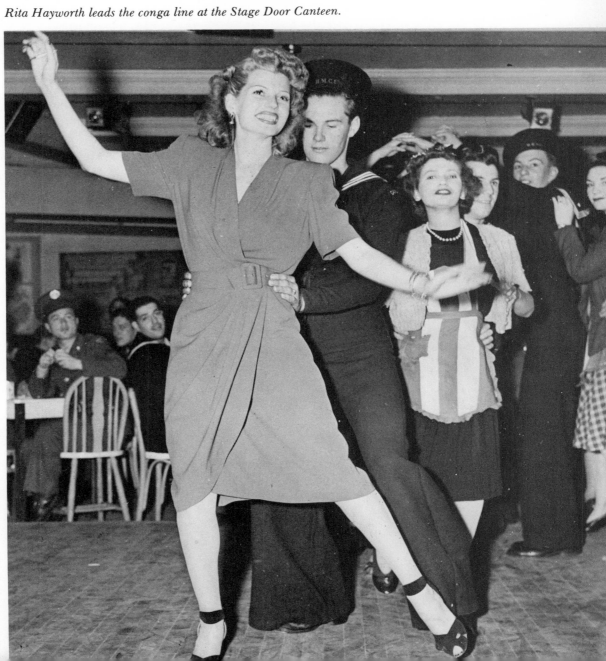

Starting with the knees flexed, the first step moved forward and straightened the leg, the second closed to the first with a slight flex, and the third movement was to straighten both legs in place with a little mark-time step. The rhythm was slow, quick, slow and the upper body had a slight undulating roll. The pattern of the movement traveled around the floor but did not gobble up space the way jitterbugging did; and besides samba dancers did not hazard life and limb.

Throughout the history of social dancing there have been "spot" and "traveling" dances, that is, those which require participants to remain pretty much in place during the dance and those which require them to utilize lots of space. At the turn of the century the Viennese waltz was a marathon event compared to the slower waltz forms which were as pretty to watch but were not preoccupied with traversing the dancing area quite so greedily. Nor were the rumba and samba. Americans had to learn how to move their hips in the rumba, which was pretty strange to most of them, but they could move easily to accustom themselves to the lilt of the samba. To popularize the rumba, teachers had to change it from its original Cuban form. The basic pattern, as it emerged in Cuba, was a diamond-shaped and the movement started before the beat rather than right on it. For American enjoyment, the floor plan was designed as the more familiar box and the accent shifted to the first beat. It was a compromise but at least it started the hips moving.

In Hollywood, the rage for South American entertainers brought Cesar Romero and Carmen Miranda to popular attention. He was the Latin lover and she was the lady with the towering headpieces that looked like fruitstand pyramids. A popular, catchy tune, "Brazil," was heard and that nice, bouncy Latin rhythm for the samba, rumba, and conga was provided by the bands of Xavier Cugat, Pupi Campo, Tito Puente, and Perez Prado. Conga snake lines formed whenever anyone yelled "Conga!" on the ballroom floor and the serpentine line of men and women holding the hips of the person in front would wend its one, two, three, kick, way throughout the room till it had picked up the maximum number of participants and then would just dissolve.

Of course, there was the inevitable reaction and Harold Rome wrote, *South America Take It Away,* a song imploring South America to take back all of those dances that were appearing on the regular band sets. It speculated that the originators of the dances were constructed differently in the sacroiliac and that they were just too strenuous for the North American habituated to another way of moving. It was fruitless; dances of Latin origin like the mambo, limbo, and pachanga would continue to show up. They were catching and introduced a new concept of body movement to the ballroom floor.

By the end of the war, the world had definitely changed, but it took a while for everyone to realize it. John D. Rockefeller Jr. assembled the land for the future United Nations buildings in New York with a generous $8.5 million disbursement, bebop moved into fashion in advanced jazz circles, and people started to see "flying saucers." A million young men and women enrolled in colleges under the funds provided returning veterans for their education and blacks began to appear in professional sports. Jackie Robinson starred as second baseman of the Dodgers (then the lovable Brooklyn Bums) and the globe was circled in 73 hours (and 5 minutes) by air, whereas it had taken Nelly Bly almost as many days in the gay nineties. There was an obvious air of prosperity as the money saved during the war when there was little to buy flooded the marketplace. Houses were erected with the same rapidity that "Liberty" merchant ships slid down the slipways during the war and Arthur Murray dance studios grossed $12 million in one year after the war as opposed to $2 million in the last year before it. Then came the "new" look.

Everyone was tired of wartime austerity and was hungry for glamour. Couturier Christian Dior sat down at his Parisian drawing board and dropped hemlines from thigh to ankle with a sweep of the brush. The clothes were cut with a fullness that had been absent and a curvy, feminine look to the hips was very much favored. It restored a smartness and formality to clothes that skipped back past the austerity years and attempted to reestablish contact with the chic, peacetime world of the thirties. The clothes were opulent and used cloth conspicuously and lavishly.

Entire wardrobes had to be completely discarded and replaced with the "new" look. The change that everyone was ready for had arrived. Governments plagued with shortages in all consumer goods, were not pleased and tried to discourage the "wasteful" styling in favor of trimmer clothes that used far less cloth. The effort was totally without success; women were tired of looking like "Rosie the Riveter" and yearned to be feminine again.

Musicals constructed elaborate spectacles around themes plucked from wartime experiences. James Michener's *Tales of the South Pacific* provided the plot for *South Pacific* which featured Navy nurse Mary Martin singing and washing "That Man Right Out of My Hair" each night, and included the velvet-voiced operatic bass Ezio Pinza as a French planter in the islands. *Call Me Mister* expressed the desire of every conscripted man. Irving Berlin returned with *Annie Get Your Gun,* and Cole Porter's *Kiss Me Kate* made sophisticated slapstick out of Shakespeare. The "Carousel Waltz" emerged from *Carousel,* while *High Button Shoes, Brigadoon,* and *Finnian's Rainbow* provided enough tunes to start any idle feet tapping. *Ballet Ballads,* the first musical carried primarily by dancing rather than acting, made its appearance and Mae West successfully revived *Diamond Lil* just to let everyone know that she was still around.

There was inflation, there was an increasingly intense "cold" war between East and West in Europe, but there wasn't any shooting and the boys were home and anxious to make up for lost time. The country went on a two-decade economic spree, feeling that it had earned the right to enjoy itself after the Depression and the privations of wartime.

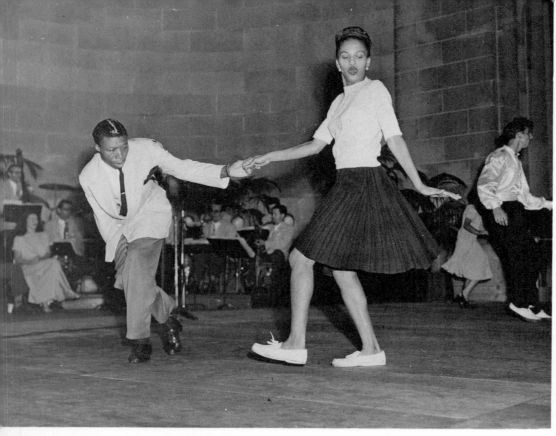

*The male half
of a jitterbugging couple
regards his partner's feet
with admiration.*

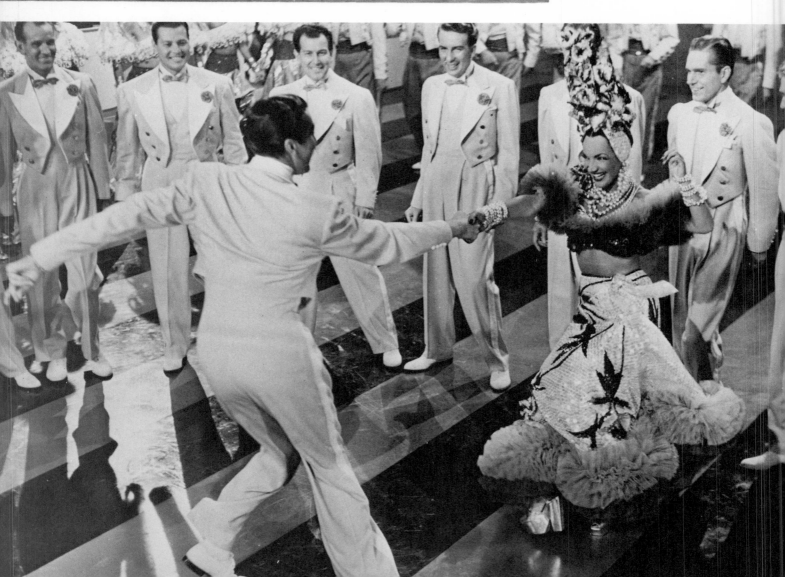

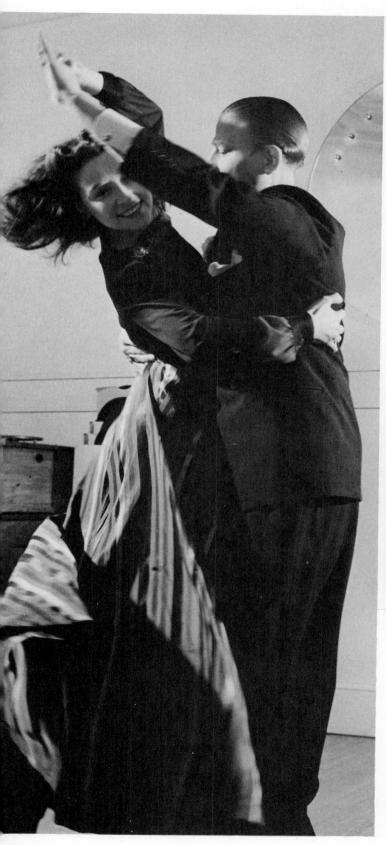

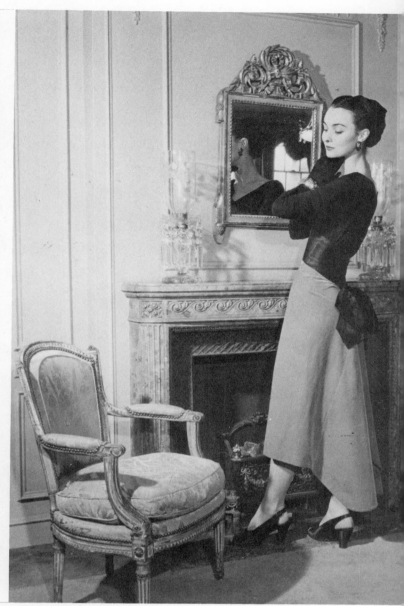

The "New Look" in fashion.

Studio demonstration of the samba.

e Latin touch with Cesar Romero and Carmen Miranda.

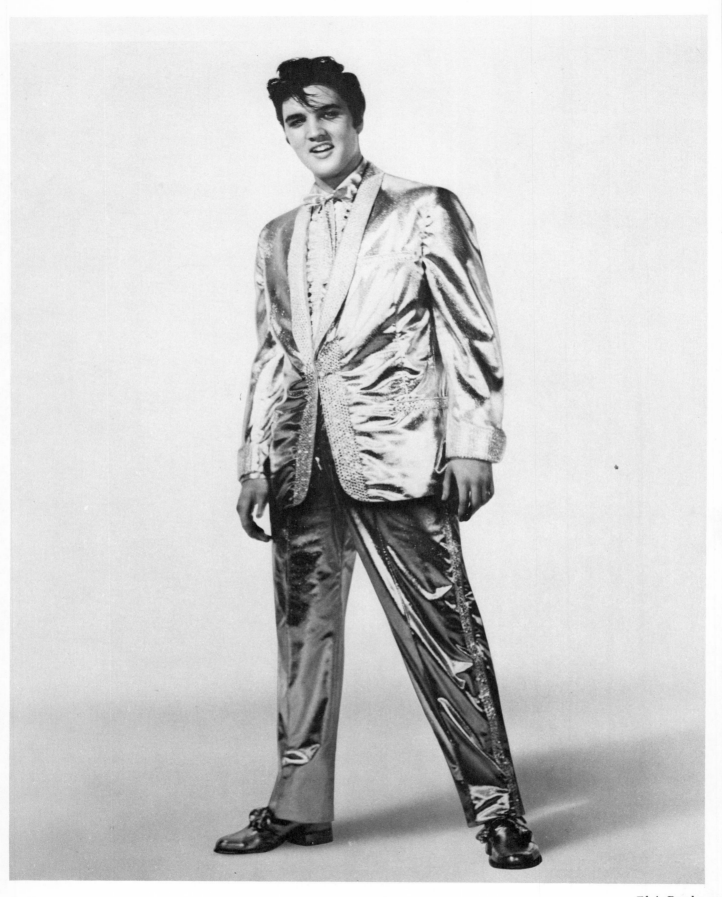

Elvis Presley

1950-1959

It was a decade of transition when old customs, dances, and music began to give way to younger, less traditional forms. Television came of age as the most popular form of mass entertainment and veteran Frank Sinatra could cut a goldie record as well as newcomer Elvis Presley.

COOLTIME

Elvis Presley was just into his teens and decidedly unknown when the decade started. By the time he entered the service toward its end, it was as if the army had drafted an entire musical movement. Like any good old boy from Memphis he heeded his country's induction notice, but unlike others he recorded two years' worth of tunes so that the incredible momentum he had generated as the most infamous rock 'n' roller might not be lost while he was away.

The young man with the slightly greasy hair, the pouty lips that had the trance of a sneer, and startling clothes ranging from leather to lamé caused offense in moralistic circles, not for what he sang so much as for the way he sang it. Shortly after he first came to public notice with goldies "Don't Be Cruel" and "Love Me Tender," he was nicknamed "Elvis the Pelvis". The public was dying to see him, having heard the rumors of his "obscene" gyrations, and the program director of the Ed Sullivan variety show wanted to present him. The problem was how to telecast something "suggestive" on family television. The solution was to show half of Elvis, the upper half, and let him sing away. People's curiosity was only partially satisfied, however, and it wasn't long before the whole singer was shown on the television screen.

Elvis had a provocative roll to the hips which hadn't been seen outside of the more obscure black clubs; the public which had been brought up on nice well-behaved singers delivering the more traditional ballads that had ruled the popular music field since the end of the First World War, was not prepared for the blatant sensual suggestiveness of Mr. Presley. He was functioning as a conduit for black musical energy and translating it for a white audience as musicians had been doing all along. The music business had a special category, rhythm and blues, that kept track of the best sellers among black musicians and audiences. There was a covert racism here that wasn't dissipated until the term rock 'n' roll came into popular usage. Following the lead of radio disc jockey Alan Freed, all singers employing the style were treated equally by the rating charts. Just the same, the older generation regarded rock 'n' roll with disdain, and the early variety, contemptuously referred to as "bubblegum" rock by a later, acidic, Vietnam war generation, was defiantly kid music. It reveled in not being sophisticated and in not being grown up.

The beat was simple, primitive; one might contend that the sound was sweet. The lyrics worried over such dilemmas as whether the object of love would still remember the adorer after summer vacation and they were sung and consumed by virtual children. Elvis was relatively old at a time when sub-teens had hits. They didn't care about jazz and they certainly didn't care about the sort of world that could put "The Tennessee Waltz" at the top of the best seller list. That was for the old folks and so was their kind of dancing. Something new was needed and it emerged, of all places, in staid Philadelphia which was still holding "The Assembly" ball each year as it had done since 1748. The forum was "American Bandstand," to which kids were invited to dance and give their opinions of new releases, meet the artists, and, with the start of telecasting in 1956, to reach audiences estimated at 20 million daily. The host was a genial young man named Dick Clark who genuinely seemed happy to be there and to enjoy the kids. Clark was well dressed, in jacket and tie, as were all the kids who flocked to be part of the show.

They did a variety of dances, one of which the most popular was the Stroll. Customarily four couples faced one another, with the boys comprising one column and the girls the other. The basic pattern, as the dance developed, was like that of the country-style Virginia reel, but it was done with greater deliberateness and an emphasis on being "cool." In unison the two lines would cross one foot in front of the other while stepping sideways, taking six steps in one direction, then crossing the other foot in back and returning to the starting point. The boy and girl at the head of the two files then grasped hands, walked, did half turns as they strolled down the center of the lines, and separated to take their places at the foot of their respective columns. After each of the couples had taken this little stylish saunter, all the boys and girls returned to the facing lines and repeated the unison sidesteps, throwing in some half turns. The Stroll covered a certain amount of ground but the Creep was almost rooted in place. It was done by individual couples who faced one another in the standard social dance position. But there was a distinct slump to the posture and the slow shuffling movement that they employed to move backward and forward made a turtle look like a speedster. The effort of moving seemed almost too much for the participants who were decidedly "cool" in their approach to dancing. They danced but their attitude implied that it almost wasn't worth the effort.

While this activity went on in plain view of the television audience, that same audience was being bombarded by a variety of other images, some highly contrasted. First there was "Uncle Miltie," and then there was "Uncle Fultie." Milton Berle had earned himself the title of "Mr. Television" as well, because back in the early days of the medium he had been the first major comedian and variety entertainer to tailor a show specially for the medium. There weren't that many sets in the late forties and early fifties and people that had them found friends and neighbors dropping in Tuesday evening to watch "Uncle Miltie."

The proud owners, who had paid a stiff price for the novel machine, started to complain that it wasn't the purchase price of the set that hurt them but the expense of entertaining with drinks and snacks. Anyone with access to a television set did not stir from it on Tuesday evening. Social gatherings and club meetings were shifted so as not to conflict with the telecast. It was a striking demonstration of the attention-getting potential of the gleaming cathode tube.

Three years after "Uncle Miltie", Monsignor, later Bishop, Fulton J. Sheen mesmerized audiences with a weekly half-hour sermon on the ways of God. Berle humorously dubbed him "Uncle Fultie" but wasn't entirely pleased when Sheen's highly rated show was placed in competition with his own for a while. Sheen's darkly glittering eyes seemed to bore into a viewer with an intensity that was almost measurable. With chalk and blackboard he demonstrated just how the overall scheme of things worked and he was followed avidly by his millions of adoring fans. Uncles "Miltie" and "Fultie" were both genuine media heavyweights. Later, when rock dancing made it to the airwaves, it too really took off. Even young, nursing mothers sat fascinated and became familiar with the regulars on "American Bandstand," like Justine (Corelli) and Kenny (Rossi) who, like Louis from South Philly, were widely known by their first names.

If "American Bandstand" held the younger set in thrall, Arthur Murray and his wife and partner Kathryn held the older set's attention with their telecast "party" which combined stories, demonstrations, and celebrity dance contests. All generations were dancing but they were dancing to different beats. The adults favored the perennial favorites, the fox-trot

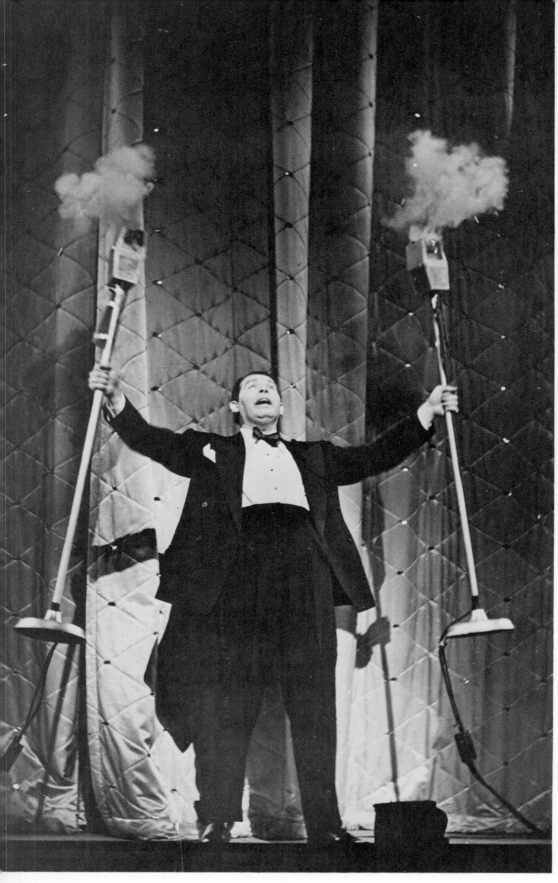
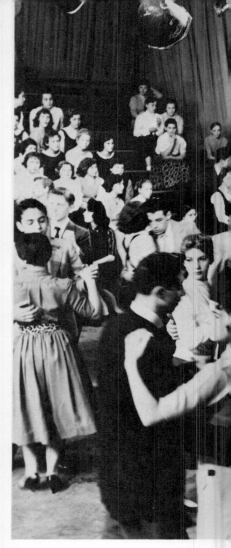

"Mr. Television," Milton Berle, known affectionately as "Uncle Miltie."

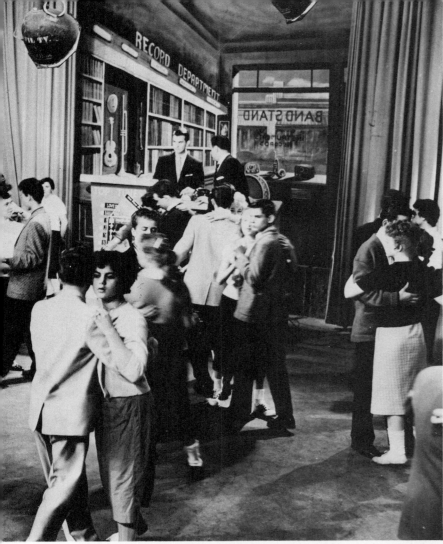

On the dance floor at
"American Bandstand."

M.C. Dick Clark holds up
a new release on "American Bandstand."

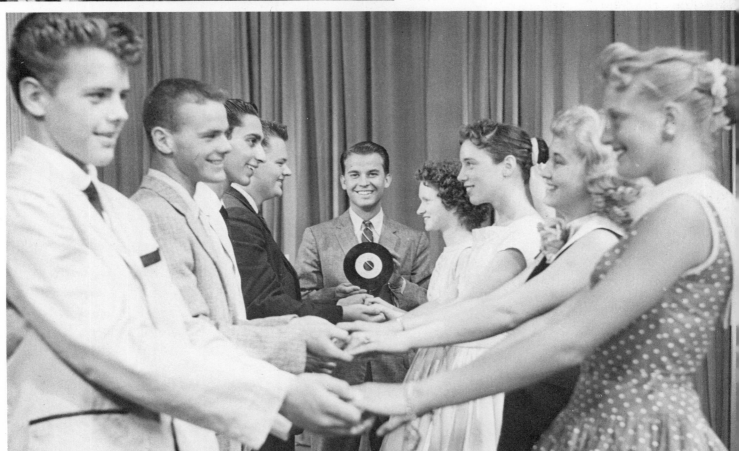

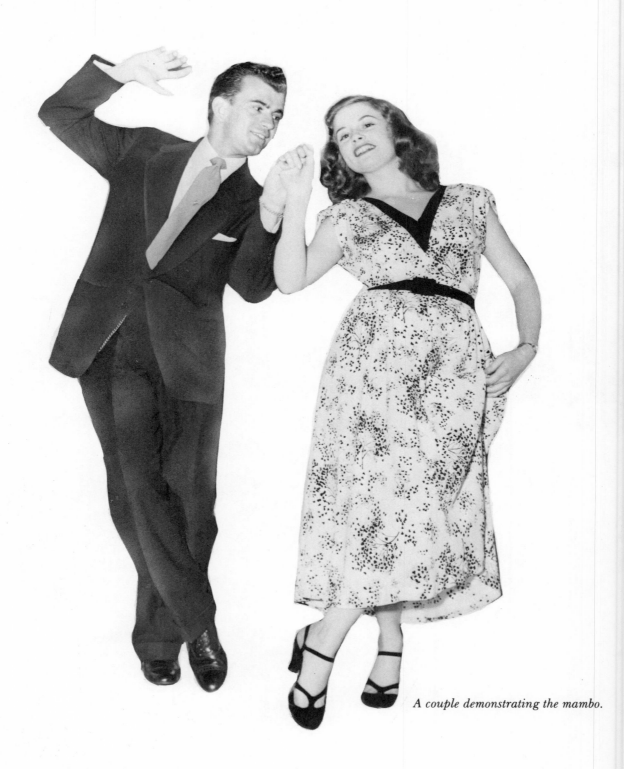

A couple demonstrating the mambo.

and the waltz with whatever was the latest Latin dance. The mambo, which had made its appearence in the previous decade was a fiendishly difficult dance for the general public. It was of Cuban origin but unlike the rumba had not been adapted for the American audience. It was a combination of jazz andLatin rhythm requiring anticipatory movements that were strange to North Americans and an active torso that had the sort of sassy lilt they were just not accustomed to.

There was a great sense of relief when the cha-cha showed up. It, too, had a Cuban origin, but its easily grasped two steps forward and three to the side made it much more accessible to non-Latins. It was more languid in its pacing and the little triple shuffle of the feet was decidedly catchy. The cha-cha obliterated the mambo in no time. The tempo was highly adaptable and even old tunes like "Tea for Two" could be turned into the cha-cha quite readily. The dancing public was moving in two different directions simultaneously, although the tensions between the older and younger generations were not ideologically expressed as they would be in a few years.

It was the time of the Korean War, which was officially designated a United Nations "police action," and the post-World War II generation marched off to it with scarcely a murmur. There were few demonstrations and annoyance was expressed privately to friends, not publicly. The country had become aware of a generation of writers who called themselves "Beat" and who announced that the times were out of joint. Their grammatical looseness prompted one establishment stylist, Truman Capote, to label what they wrote "typing," not "writing." The Beat generation's writing reflected their sense of oppression by a society which was strangling on rules and regulations and, not being responsive to problems of a deeper nature that were threatening the individual. Not even Elvis, the obvious rebel, heeded. He donned olive drab like everyone else when he received his draft notice.

The musical world was also in a transitional state. Though rock 'n' roll was on the march, Frank Sinatra, Perry Como, Jimmy Dorsey, and Pat Boone cut best sellers that were in the Top Ten even after Elvis had sold over three million records. The decade had hits like "Shrimp Boats" from Jo Stafford, "Come-on-a-My-House" by Rosemary Clooney, Teresa Brewer's "Music, Music, Music," Peggy Lee's "Lover," and Kay Starr's "Wheel of Fortune." Frankie Laine, Vic Damone, and Harry Belafonte churned out hits and the Mills Brothers scored again with their mellow renditions of old standards like "Paper Doll."

Other strong sounds were being heard more frequently. The heavy piano fingers of "Fats" Domino and Jerry Lee Lewis were part and parcel of the driving beat also used by Bill Haley and The Comets. Little groups sprang up continually. The long, gradual buildup was a thing of the past and the overnight sensation appeared in the persons of The Chords, The Four Aces, Ricky Nelson, The Diamonds, Frankie Avalon, Paul Anka, Neil Sedaka, The Platters, and the Everley Brothers. The artists and recording

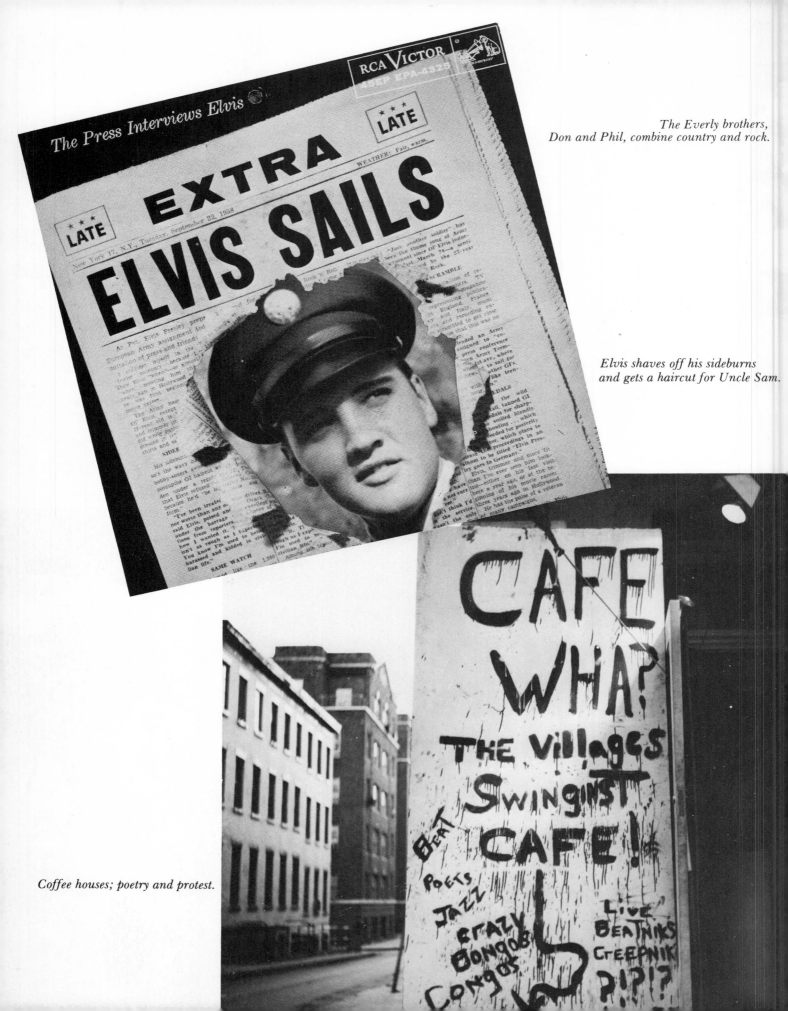

The Press Interviews Elvis

RCA Victor
45EP EPA-4325

EXTRA
ELVIS SAILS

*The Everly brothers,
Don and Phil, combine country and rock.*

*Elvis shaves off his sideburns
and gets a haircut for Uncle Sam.*

Coffee houses; poetry and protest.

CAFE
WHA?
THE Villages
SWINGInST
BEAT
CAFE!
POETS
JAZZ
CRAZY
BONGOS
CONGOS
LIVE
BEATNIKS
CREEPNIK
PIP!?

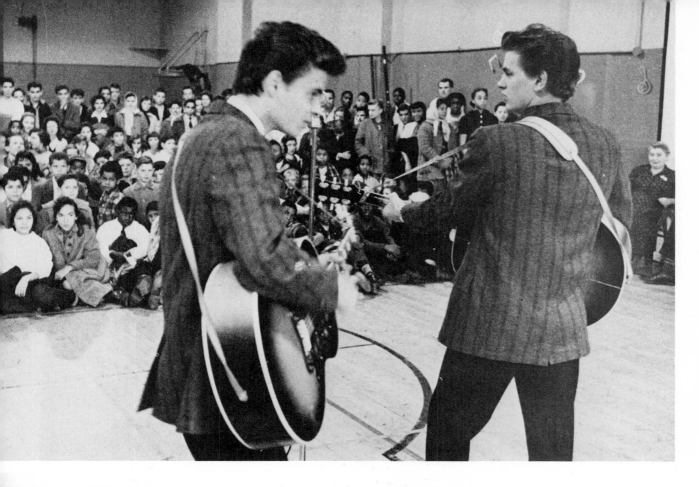

The Frug makes its appearance.

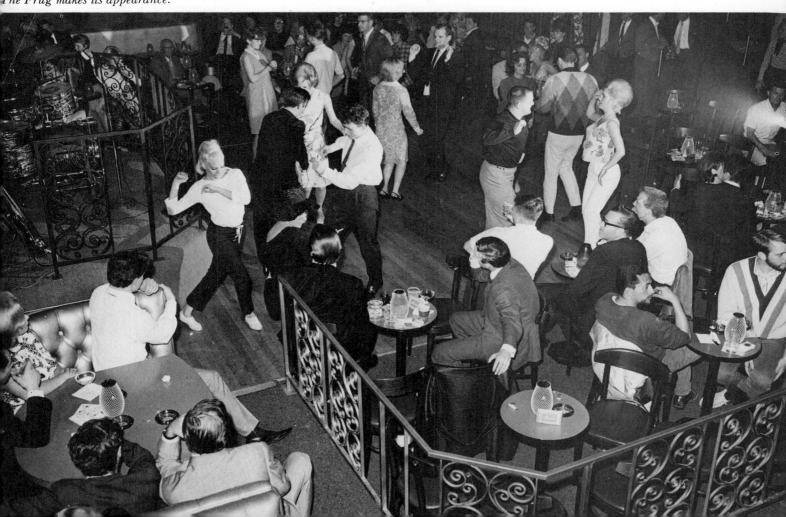

executives ruled the roost and whim could turn anyone into a rock star. They found Fabian hanging out on a stoop in Philadelphia, dubbed him "The Fabulous One," since he looked so perfect, and launched another career. That many of these performers were commercially created with electronic wizardry was proven every week on "American Bandstand" where they would come to plug their records and were under strict orders to lip-synchronize to a recorded track, rather than spoil the illusion by singing live.

On Broadway, the shows continued to spawn songs that were demanding and recognizably adult. Rogers and Hammerstein produced *The King and I,* Lerner and Lowe created *My Fair Lady,* Feuer and Martin transformed a factory production line into *The Pajama Game* and Adler and Russo made baseball the amusing starting point of *Damn Yankees.* Hollywood snapped them all up and made highly successful movies. Just to keep the kids happy, the studios signed up Elvis and churned out one formula movie after another like *Jailhouse Rock* and *Loving You* which wisely made no demands on his acting ability but racked up handsome profits from the kids who only wanted to see and hear him sing.

He was petulant, rebellious and just the sort of person that parents wouldn't approve of. He was unbuttoned in a world that was tightly buttoned down. Elvis didn't care and neither did the adoring fans who mobbed his concerts to swagger and demonstrate their "cool." They were breaking the rules that governed the old folks' world.

Newspaper columnists found in the situation a well of endless examples of new and conspicuously outrageous behavior. The mature generation didn't understand the encompassing pleasure of rock music. To older ears it sounded chaotic and it all sounded the same: loud! They missed the sophistication of mature lyricists and occasionally, to drive home their point seized on obvious nonsense but cleverly constructed songs and made them fad hits, like Perry Como's "What Did Delaware."

The kids didn't really care what the lyrics said, they liked the throbbing beat which needed full volume to achieve its aural embrace. Rock music was felt more than listened to and tended to push the hearer into a private world. Conversation was impossible on the dance floor and the kids were becoming dangerously independant of one another, frequently separating to do their individual movements. By implication they were dangerously independent of the society which had always seen dancing as a form of social relationship. The social contract itself had begun to be questioned and women were moving out of the harem of dependency that had characterized their position in society. The Philly Dog began to show up on "American Bandstand" with its back-and-forth shuffling and snapping fingers that indicated a certain heedlessness for anyone outside the dancer's own world. The emphasis was shifting away from the socially approved couple to extreme preoccupation with the individual.

At the beginning of the decade, life was not at all that way. Women were emerging, but Paris couturiers were never more powerful than at the start

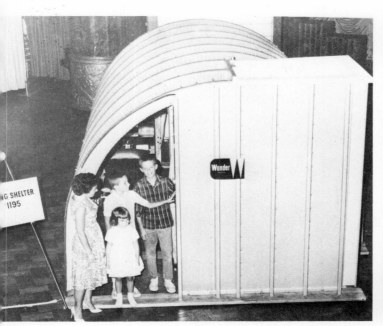 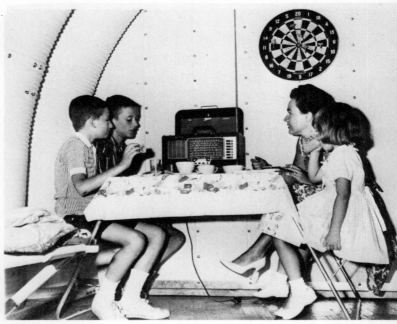

What the well-equipped fallout shelter should have.

of the fifties and women all over the fashionable world took their cue from what well dressed Parisiennes wore. They wore clothes that reflected a certain formality and featured a tailored look, and hats were accompanied by gloves. The hem had risen but stayed well below the knee. The stiletto heel was favored. There was a brief flurry of popularity for the "sack" dress, which was cut so that it bagged like a sack at the waist. It was the subject of considerable ridicule and died a quick death.

Women were highly conscious of coordinated colors when choosing cosmetics, and there was a chicness to the way they dressed. Hair was long, with a bouncy, turned-up look until the curly, curly poodle cut made its appeerence. Women looked trim; they kept curves under control with tight slimming garments, though it was considered distinctly advantageous to have a prominent bosom. The womanly, sophisticated image was the one striven for.

As the decade wore on, American women occupied more and better jobs and began to make inroads into the executive suites that had been firmly closed to all but a very few of them. The country was beset by a spasm of political anxieties involving Communists and communist activity which was fed by the actual Cold War and opportunistic use of it by ambitious politicians. The H-bomb made its frightening debut, and people talked about fallout shelters and began to stock food and water in case of an atomic attack. The Soviet Union demonstrated a large lead in space technology by launching a space satellite, "Sputnik," that circled the globe. In the midst of prosperity, there was anxiety about the future. Things seemed to be slipping slightly out of control. By the end of the decade, the slim, mature look had lost favor and a new emphasis on youth emerged. It was considered much more attractive to look like a kid. The adult world was in a mess.

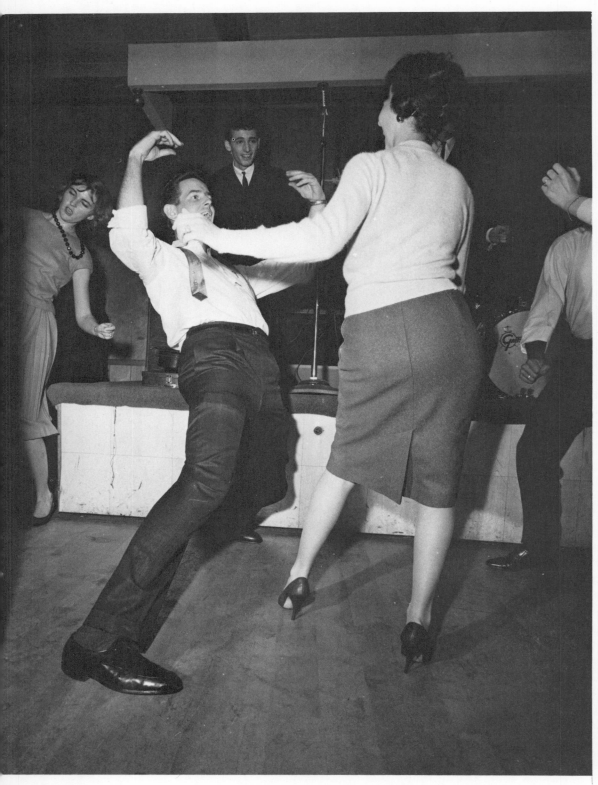

Doing the Twist at the most fashionable spot, the Peppermint Lounge.

The generation gap set old (over 30), against
young (under 30), in music, politics, and sexual freedom.
"Doin' your own thing" became the alternate life-style and on
the dance floor it meant that no one touched.

SOLO TIME

Right from the beginning of the decade, youth was the keynote. A bright, boyish president was in the White House, calling on the nation's youth to join his work, to become Peace Corps Volunteers or Volunteers in Service to America (VISTA). By the end of the decade, youth was still in the spotlight, but by then, idealistic young people had given way an alienated group of disenchanted hippies, yippies, and war protesters. The Vietnam war raged, assassinations at home had killed off three of the country's most charismatic leaders, and kids were listening to the beat of a new national anthem—a star-spangled freakout sung by Jimi Hendrix at Woodstock in 1969. It was a tumultous ten years from Camelot to cataclysm and in the beginning at least much of its energy focused on music and dance. For about six years, America became the "Land of a Thousand Dances."

The revolution actually started back in 1959, when black kids originated a dance to go along with a rising new hit record by Hank Ballard, "The

Twist." But it took another year or two and a re-recording by Chubby Checker (an ex-chicken plucker whose real name is Ernest Evans) for the dance to reach American Bandstand and the white audience. Then there was just no stopping it. America's teenyboppers saw Bandstand favorites Justine and Bob and Kenny and Arlene, doing the twist, and were soon twisting right along at home. Schools frowned on the hip-swiveling gyrations on the dance floor, but this only made twisting even more exciting and along came the limbo twist (a sort of twisting-under-the-limbo-pole dance), the slow twist and numerous variations.

Dance had very definitely taken a new turn. For one thing, adults who had been tapping their feet under the table for years, discovered that they could actually do this new dance. It was simple to learn as soon as one realized that the basic spiral movements of the hips and toros went together. The body twists first to the left as the left knee twists inward. A weight shift to the other foot and the same grinding motion of the ball of the foot is repeated as if one were actually snuffing out a cigarette but. For variety, a little kick is added now and then. The arms are kept up close to the chest, punching out and pulling back with the corresponding twists of the body. Twist partners danced independently. For the first time since the Charleston, there was plenty of room for individual expression because the partners were no longer confined to the traditional social dance position. Twist partners didn't touch and didn't depend on each other to complement their individual steps. Later variations of the twist all adhered to this new convention.

The Peppermint Lounge on West Forty-Fifth Street in New York City, once a seedy hangout of pimps and prostitutes, was responsible for turning adults on to the dance of the kids' world. "The Peppermint Twist," a hit song, originated there and catapulted the club into the headlines. Almost overnight, it became the twist headquarters of the jet set. Twisting right along came Elizabeth Taylor, Richard Burton, Jayne Mansfield, Judy Garland, and a host of others. While Joey Dee and The Starlighters were grinding out the music, their stellar older audience was twisting the night away on the dance floor. If anyone wanted private lessons, "Killer" Joe Piro was around to introduce them to the subtleties of the Loco-Motion, which featured groups of eight in circles starting up and accelerating like a train, or the Mashed Potatoes, with its heel swivels and any number of other twist spin-offs.

The dance had arrived and the press gave it plenty of coverage. Along with the twist and all the variations and successors, almost simultaneously came two imports from Europe: the discothèque from France and, from England, four Liverpudlians, The Beatles. The new discos provided the place, The Beatles and those they inspired made the music, and the twist and its offspring were the dances.

The discothèque craze began in Paris but swept like wildfire through the United States. Canned music was played almost non-stop; live music for dancing was phased out except for formal occasions. As discos developed, they became more and more elaborate, offering live entertainment in the form of go-go dancers who undulated in suspended cages, on platforms, or in recessed niches, twisting and moving to the loud new rock beat. The man who presided over the selection of records played his audience like an old-fashioned dancing master calling the tune.

In New York City, discos flourished and were filled to overflowing any night of the week. At Sybil, Arthur, which was owned by Richard Burton's ex-wife, Sybil, Ondine, II Mio, The Dom, Hippopotamus, L'Interdit and dozens of other clubs, for a cover charge and the price of a drink or two, people were dancing madly, with wild enthusiasm. "Smooth" dancing—the waltzes, fox-trots, rumbas, and sambas—almost vanished in the fever for the bobbing, ducking, thrusting dances that comprised the regular disco fare. And of course, with disco dancing, no bodies touched.

In little more than a year after the first flowering of the twist, just when Chubby Checker was singing "Let's twist again like we did last summer," the dance had been turned inside out, upside down and spawned all manner of variations. It was a time of laughter and the more ridiculous the dance the better it was liked, at least for the moment. When the old comic strip "Batman" was turned into a pop television series, almost immediately a dance called the Batman appeared. Overhand strokes added to the basic twist produced the Swim, while a tugging motion as if hauling oneself hand over hand up a rope was called the Monkey. In England, an ex-milkman, Freddie Garrity, formed a band with a few of his pals and called it Freddie and the Dreamers. Freddie sang and hopped wildly up and down in front of the group and thus was born the Freddie. When asked to describe its basic movement, Freddie replied, "You have to lift up your feet like a farmer in boots coming out of a muddy field." A French photographer, Jacques Bostel, sank to the floor of a Paris discothèque after tripping and soon the whole house was hitting the deck and not long after that, La Bostella, as it was inevitably known, made its way to American dance floors.

In the early sixties there was just no end to the new dances. Many, like the Batman, Freddie, and Watusi, faded as quickly as they rose. Others lasted only as long as a hit record such as "The Fish," "The Bristol Stomp," "Popeye," and "The Hitchiker." Dances were made up in the disco for just one evening to be forgotten the next. The Pony, Fly, Madison and almost countless others came and went. The twist itself became very passé by mid-sixties, especially among the kids when the adults started dancing it and when it started appearing on the staid old formal dance floors. Two of its successors—the frug and the jerk—hung around until late in the decade. The frug began at Syracuse University and, like the twist, it was a spot dance; it didn't travel and the partners didn't touch. It too was a hip-swiveling dance, though involving more side to side motion. The hands played an important part and the common hand movement was the frug swing, which alternately brought the curved arm up from hip level to halfway across the chest and back again. Wagging the index finger in a scolding gesture was frequent as was the open palm as if asking for a

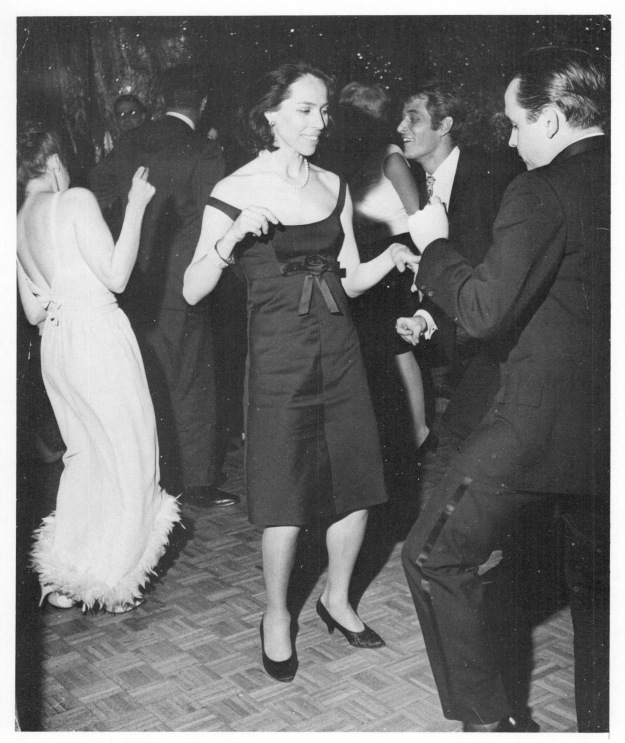

Even ballerinas were doing it.
Here Maria Tallchief of the New York City Ballet twists with companion Robert Larkin.

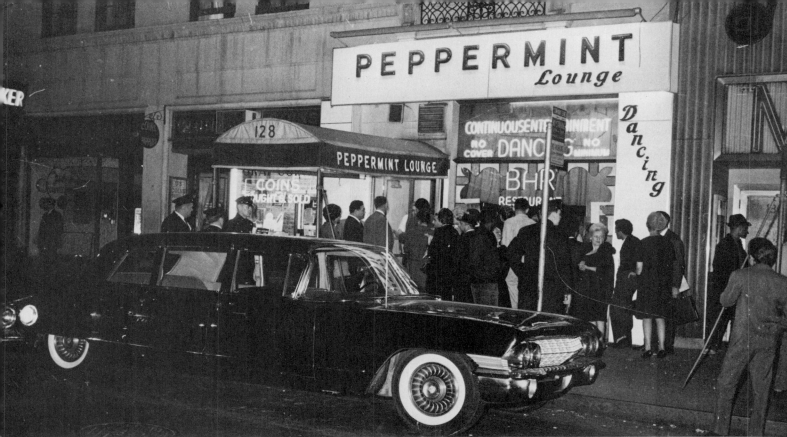

The seedy ambiance of the Peppermint Lounge
didn't deter the limousine crowd.

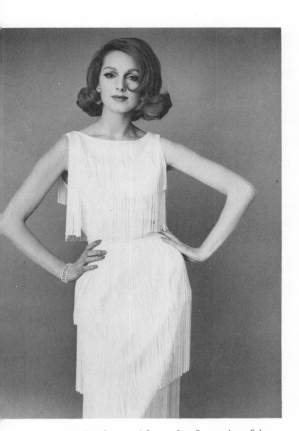

A twist dress with yards of swaying fringe.

It was about as close as anyone had to get
in those no-touch days.

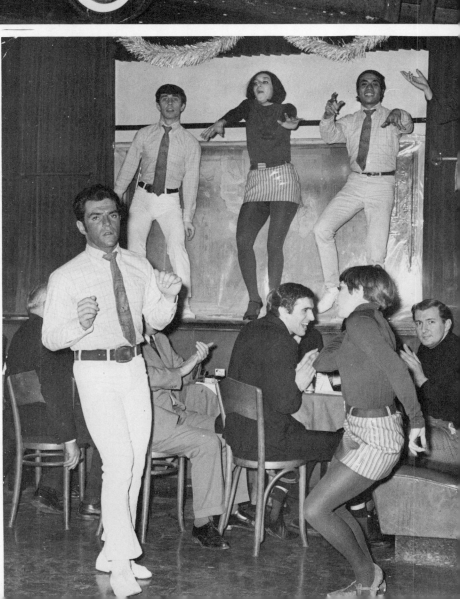

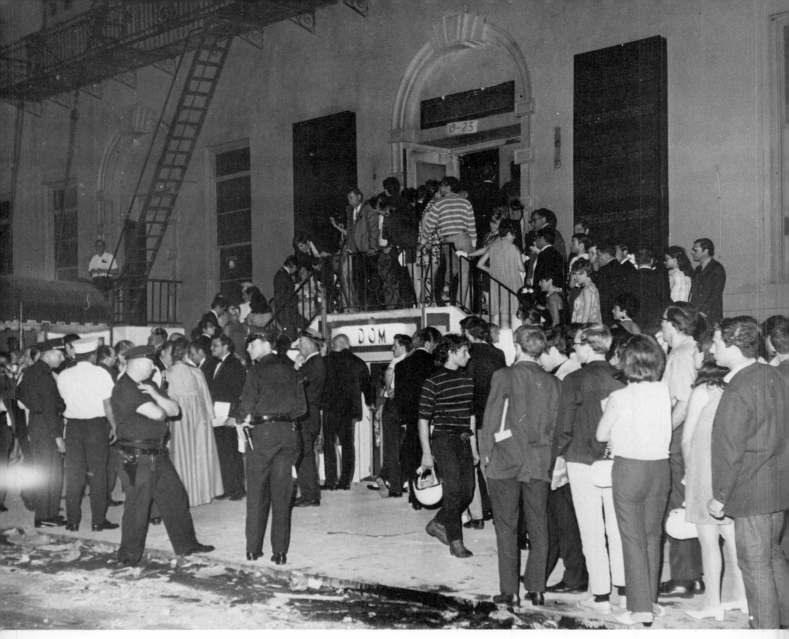

The even seedier ambiance of The Dom on the lower East Side attracted overflow crowds. Later painter Andy Warhol turned the place into The Exploding Plastic Inevitable.

handout. To do the jerk, one hand is held over the body which is snapped as the hand quickly descends. The dancer jerks with alternating hands. The jerk made its debut in 1964 with a song by the Larks and, says Dick Clark in *Rock, Roll and Remember,* "From then until the seventies the dances ceased to have names."

A few of the discos, such as Cheetah and the Electric Circus, had continued to offer live music along with canned fare. They were also taking the discothèque in a brand new direction. Designed to thrill dancers and watchers alike—and there were more and more on the sidelines as the drug culture took hold—there were fantastic psychedelic effects, strobe lights, mirrors, films, and light shows, which, with the music and dance, made the disco a total sensory experience of sight, sound, and movement.

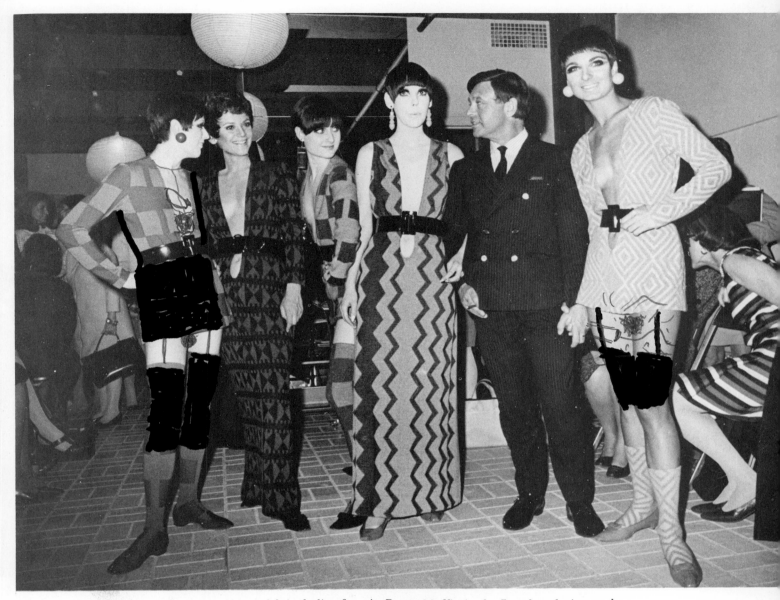

Designer Rudi Gernreich and a covey of his models including favorite Peggy Moffitt in the floor-length zig-zag dress.

The idea of crossing lines from one discipline to another was very appealing in the Age of Aquarius. One of the most ambitious of these new mega-discos was "Murray the K's World," in an abandoned hangar at Roosevelt Field, Long Island, where forty years previously, Charles Lindbergh had taken off on his solo hop to Le Bourget Airport in Paris. It featured good rock, big sound, and slide and film projections by a group of artists calling themselves USCO. They included respected moviemakers and light designers who were interested in the multimedia scene presented by rock. Disc jockey Murray (the "K") Kaufman may have grown up listening to the voice of Frank Sinatra, but he became the unparalleled and outspoken maestro of rock in the mid-sixties, who boasted that he was the "Fifth Beatle," responsible for their discovery in America. On his radio show, at a time when commercials were overwhelmingly frequent, he would announce three uninterrupted plays as a "triple ripple," hit records over a year old were "blasts from the past" and to loyal fans who knew the answers to Murray's musical quizzes he would send a "submarine race watching shirt." He even had his own language, a sort of fast-talking version of the pig-latin of childhood. Kids loved him.

Murray the K wasn't the only one to become personally involved in the

"Killer" Joe Piro steps out with Carol Channing.

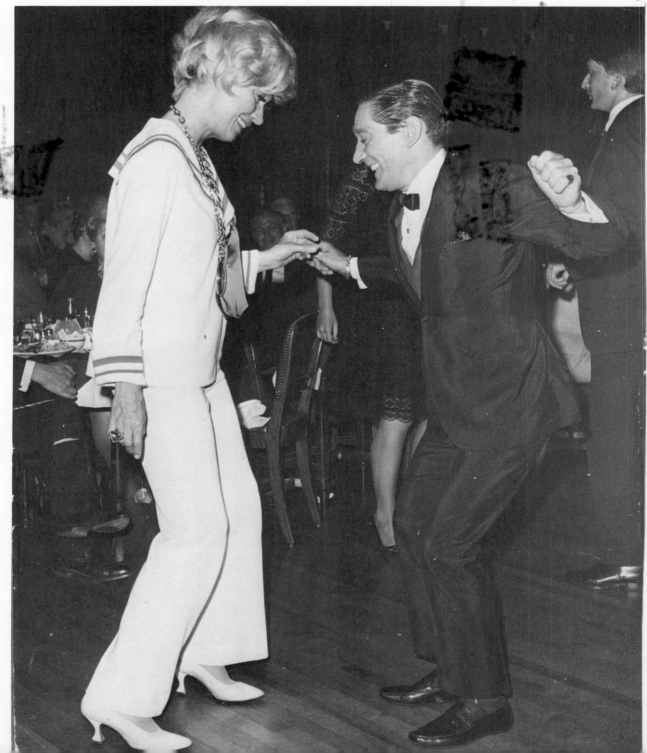

disco world. Rock and rock dancing turned up everywhere; even the halls of the Metropolitan Museum reverberated with a rock beat during a wild opening party, while downtown, pop-artist Andy Warhol, associated with soup cans and superstars, decided to buy his own discothèque. He dubbed it "The Exploding Plastic Inevitable" and packed it with a far-out assortment of friends and visitors.

Dress codes had disappeared in all but the most stodgy places. The

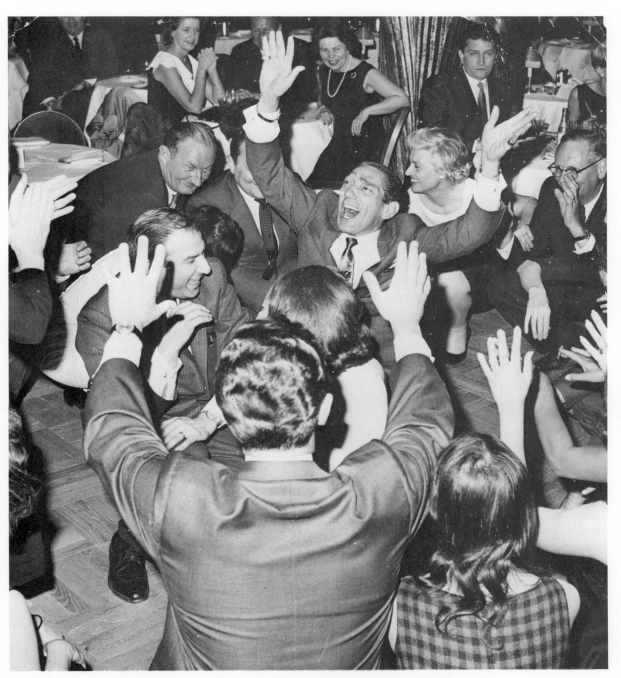

"Killer" Joe introduces "La Bostella" to the United States after its triumphs abroad.

unusual was in and the more extravagant the costume, the more successful it was. Everyone began to dress like rock stars. White Courrèges boots, wraparound glasses, plastic and paper clothing, body jewelery and body painting, wide bell-bottom pants, topless bathing suits, long fringed jackets, miniskirts, maxiskirts—one fad followed another in rapid succession.

The little girl look was in. Hair went bouffant for a while although lots of women just wore it straight. Hair coloring offered all sorts of interesting alternatives to nature's original gift; women decided what color pleased them most and went ahead and colored their hair without any concern about what anyone else might think. The stigma had been removed from this most dramatic cosmetic exercise. In the fifties the first major hair coloring push was instigated with a wifely (wedding ring in view), motherly (child or husband in background), woman looking straight into the camera with the provocative headline, "Does she or doesn't she?" The ad went on to state that only her hairdresser knew for sure. The fact is that even if she didn't, the idea had been planted and the hair coloring business enjoyed excellent sales for the remainder of the decade. Any hesitation was gone by the sixties when hair coloring for men began to be advertised.

Cosmetics went to any extreme that a woman chose to use them. Clownface or close to it was not unheard of. There was a celebration of the strange and assymetrical and in a sense, ugly was beautiful. A bizarre or costume element in clothes began to manifest itself and Paris became concerned. A concerted effort was made to drop hemlines and restore the sculptured thirties look. But imposed fashion didn't elicit immediate compliance any longer and women resisted any entirely new look. Most women had come to the conclusion that there were certain styles that suited them personally and that those were the ones they wanted to hang onto, no matter what the fashion magazines or designers said. Every woman was doing her own thing!

Men, long the silent minority in matters of dress began to exhibit a concern with style. Being comfortably rumpled didn't suffice in the swingin 'sixties. So along with sideburns and longer hair, men became more daring in terms of clothes cut and coloring. While fads like the Nehru jacket left most men untouched, there was a trend toward casual colorfulness that would have been unthinkable previously.

The musical energy of the country had left Tin Pan Alley; that collection of songwriters who, for fifty years, had turned out songs that were sloppy, silly, sentimental, sophisticated, smart-alecky, serious, slick and supremely successful. The Broadway stage began to depend more and more on production values instead of tunes. The effects were dazzling, but no one went away whistling the scenery. A major exception to the rule was an off-Broadway musical called "Hair," with music by Galt MacDermot. The show was so successful in a limited run, that they polished it up and brought it to the Great White Way. A bit of nudity was seen through a veiled twilight-lit stage and people could actually hum the tunes like "Age of Aquarius." The original cast album was modestly successful but the music really took off with The Fifth Dimension's recording of two of the songs from the show. Rock had made it to the big time in the establishment theater as well as in its own new circuit of concerts, events, and celebrations.

Rock itself had undergone a drastic change. The decade had begun with such innocuous hits as "Sherry" (which was given eight counts and sung as "She-eh-eh-eh-eh-eh-ree-ee Bay-ay-bee"), or "Come Softly" (the chorus repeated "dum dum duh-um doo duh-um dooby doo"). All that had changed with the four-four beat of The Beatles. Their early music was easy to dance to and the other British groups—The Dave Clark Five, Herman's Hermits, and all the rest—followed The Beatles' example. Most of these other groups disappeared, however, after a few years. The Rolling Stones were different. They had a distinctive style and like the Beatles, they changed with the times which by 1966, had certainly changed. Everyone seemed to be turning on to drugs and kids were dropping out in droves. They headed for Haight-Ashbury in San Francisco or the East Village in New York City. These were the flower children, or hippies as they came to be known, and they sang about peace and love and lived together in communes. They followed Timothy Leary, Ken Kesey, and other gurus, experimenting with the hallucinogenic drugs especially LSD or "acid" as it was aptly nicknamed. The new drug culture inspired a new music, acid rock, which was not to be danced to. The long haired and wildly dressed audience sat back and grooved on the intricacies of their new beat with a drug-heightened sensitivity. They flocked to theatres such as Bill Graham's original Fillmore in San Francisco or the Fillmore East in New York. There and at places as diverse as Yankee Stadium, Carnegie Hall, and even the august stage of the Metropolitan Opera, the musicians performed. The Grateful Dead, the Jefferson Airplane, The Who, Janis Joplin, Jimi Hendrix and scores of others soared on stage while the audience soared in their seats.

By 1969, even the confines of the theatre were left behind altogether at the Woodstock Festival, where youth celebrated three days of peace, love, and music on a six-hundred acre farm near the little village of Woodstock, New York. With a half million people, the festival proclaimed itself a small city and enjoyed good music, dope, and company. The audience became the event and eclipsed the stars performing As for the dance at Woodstock, it was there all right and might be called such names as the Woodstock mudslide or the great rain dance or any number of things. It was a dance of life at the time; it no longer required a dance floor, partners, or a certain pattern of steps. The dancers swayed, swooped, and twirled in a formless expression of ecstacy or sometimes despair.

Individuals sank into the world of the self and hoped for the best. They were feeling their way through rather than thinking their way through. Those rocking, twisting, no-touching dances suited the times just fine. Responsibilities toward anyone else were definitely being kept to a minimum.

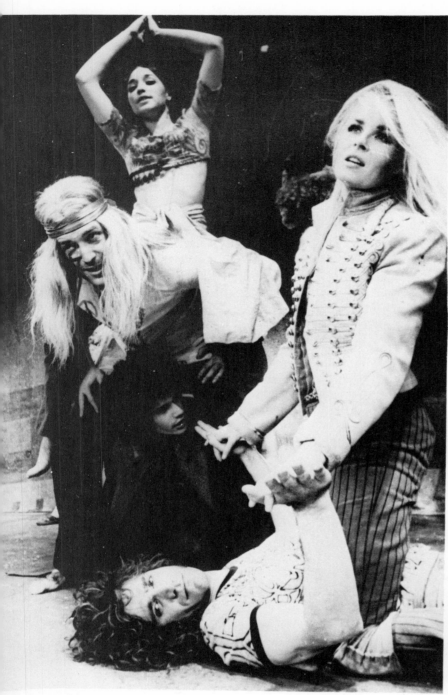

Rock makes Broadway with the production Hair.

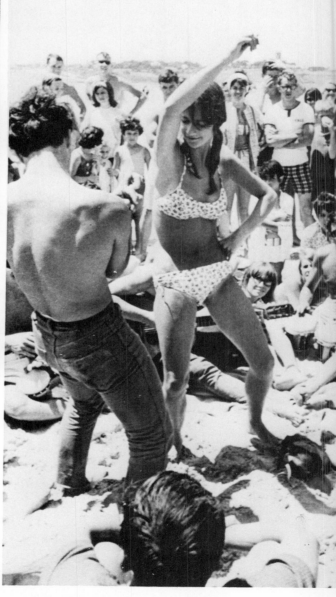

A couple on the beach do the Watusi at Newport, Rhode Island during the jazz festival.

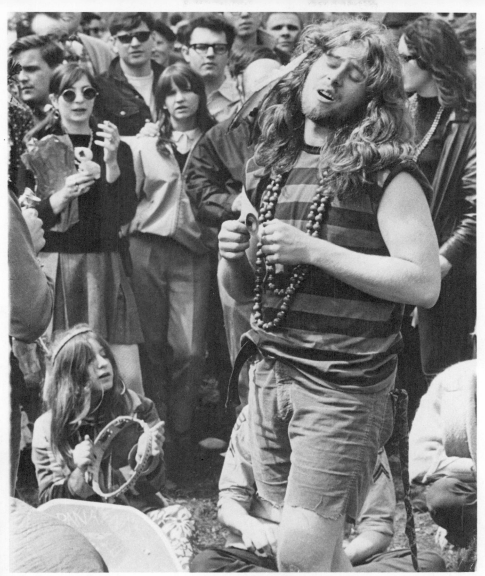

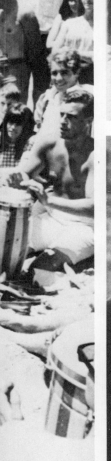

"Doing his own thing,"
in the midst of a crowd.

The Beatles: John Lennon,
Ringo Starr,
George Harrison, and
Paul McCartney
in A Hard Day's Night.

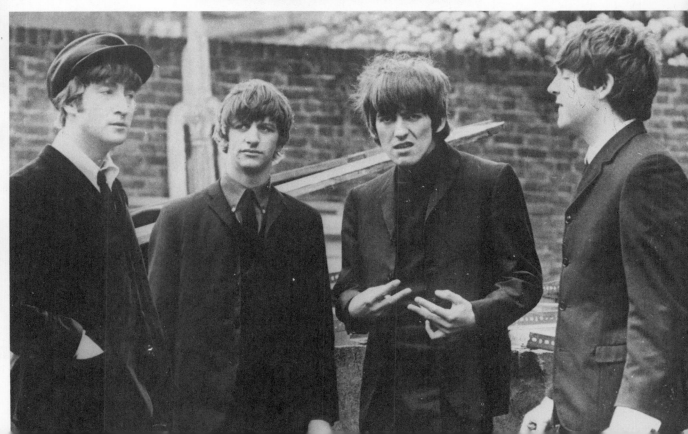

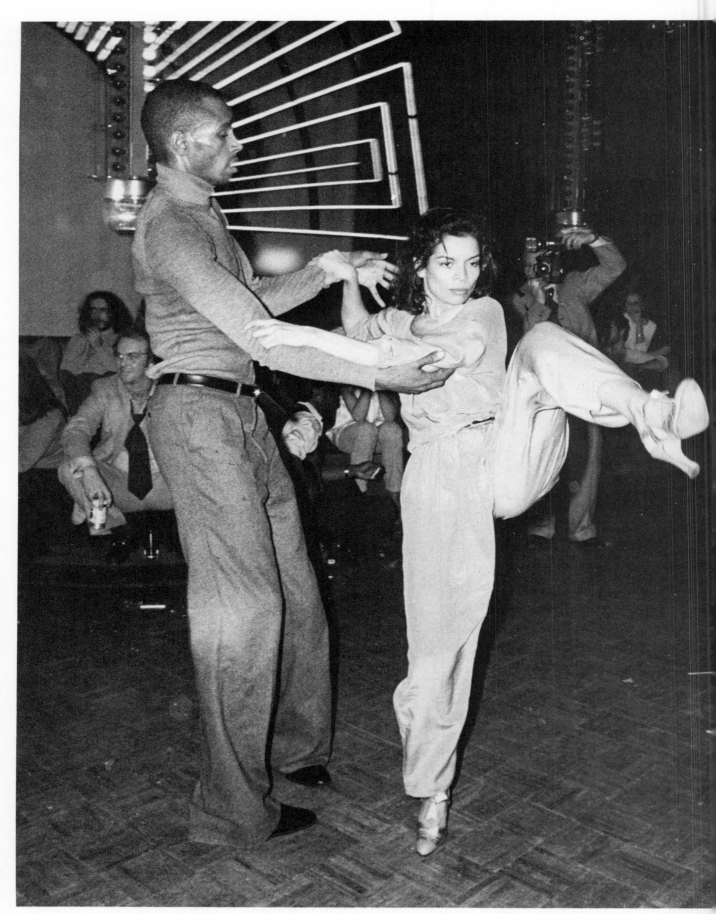

Bianca Jagger dancing with Sterling St. Jacques.

1970-1979

The wearied generations started to become reconciled
as the under 30's slipped over the dividing line
into the older camp. Institutions would never be
quite the same again but cooperation was
preferable to confrontation and doing
the Hustle joyously reunited partners on the dance floor.

SALSA

The divisive war in Vietnam finally came to a lurching halt, but not before the army had given up trying to induct ordinary citizens and had come to rely on paid volunteers. The flower children disappeared; they just seemed to wilt away after Altamont, a Rolling Stones rock festival during which a fan was brutally murdered by members of the Hell's Angels motorcycle gang. Watergate delivered a new body blow to the country, which further convulsed or perhaps exulted over President Nixon's resignation. The nation was weary and exhausted individuals turned with some relief to institutions. The college prom staged a comeback after having languished for a half-dozen years. Nostalgia swept the land. At antique sales, little plastic pens and pencils from the 1939-40 World's Fair in New York fetched precious metal prices. At one such sale, a woman was overheard whispering to another, "I told you never to throw anything away!"

The extremes of the sixties when clothing was a costume, often garish, were rejected but not the independence gained. A loose, casual look

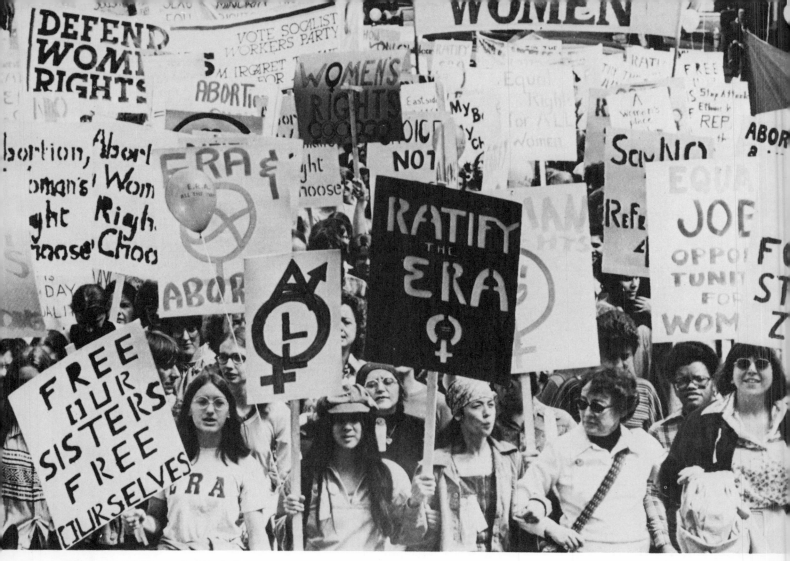

The start of "Woman's Week."

emerged that was something less than dressy but decidedly more than jeans and a top. When jeans were worn, chances were that they had a designer's label attached and had cost well over the price of a pair of Levi's. The miniskirt vanished again and hemlines could land anywhere between the ankle and knee. Hair, kept long all through the sixties, was given its first clipping of the decade and women wore curly layered hair helped along with a permanent which kept it in place without constant attention.

Rock music began to take on social issues, the kids had stopped dancing altogether and were spending time hanging out in the early seventies. Listening was in and dancing was out, with two exceptions. The old smoothies of over thirty still fox-trotted away and, in Hispanic clubs, hip young Latinos were doing an exotic new dance which came to be known as the Hustle.

Latin music had been a fact of ballroom life since the tango became the height of abandonment before the First World War. Each decade saw some new and unusual rhythm develop in the working class districts of South America or the Caribbean and then turn up in some of the smarter social milieus of the United States. The rumba, samba, cha-cha and many others had all enjoyed the limelight.

The Hustle didn't have to be imported; it emerged from El Barrio, the unfashionable blue-collar district on the northern border of Manhattan's decidedly fashionable Upper East Side. The Hustle was the first Latin dance indigenous to North America. As with other Latin dances, people touched while dancing. The Hustle was a smooth dance with an intricate trellis of turns which flowed with grace and beauty. It looked like the old Lindy-Hop smoothed out, but it was danced in six rather than four counts. Its quick footwork and aggressive stomp announced its Latin origin and the Latin Hustle often throws in one more count with all seven steps performed to six beats of the music. It's a complex dance of flying feet and the music is called *salsa.* It was all over the tiny, popular neighborhood clubs before anyone in the middle class even knew it existed.

With the hustle, discos returned to the social scene with a rush after having been ignored in favor of do-it-yourself parties anywhere and everywhere. The dance floor with its limitations was again recognized as the place for couples to meet and be together and the new danced offered a new kind of intimacy. In fact, a magazine, *Foxy Lady,* came right out and said what everyone know all along in an article titled "How to Dance Dirty." The particulars of nuzzling and rubbing had been common knowledge; now they were set down the way that rules for any social game might be. A fad dance based on Chinese martial arts called the Kung Fu made a brief appearance. For the most part it was an arm chop-and-thrust sequence that was decorative and harked back to the no-touch days of the sixties. It was too violent for new-found peace of the seventies. The Bump was another simple fad that vanished as quickly as it arrived. The couple did touch though, which was the urge-to-merge direction of the decade. Their touching in the Bump mainly consisted of strategically maneuvered brushes of the hips, pelvis and other body parts and the dance itself could easily have been illustrative material for the "How to Dance Dirty" article. Some of the dancers bruised by the Bump, may have yearned for the years of no-touch dancing.

California developed its own interesting variation on the New York Hustle. The dancers didn't touch, but they moved as a group, all kicking and stepping in unison and woe to those who moved in the wrong direction.

For the most part, disco music followed a simple formula which can take any old favorite like "Tangerine," "Baby Face," or even "Brazil" and tune it for the dance floor with the right bass rhythm, percussion, and accent. Barry White's "Love's Theme" was the orchestral version of the sound, while the Bee Gees showed the excitement a small group could generate with "Jive Talkin' " and the sound track from *Saturday Night Fever.*

By 1977, just in case anyone had missed the new dance craze, along came the movie *Saturday Night Fever.* It catapulted John Travolta into the superstar category in one sensational performance and brought disco danc-

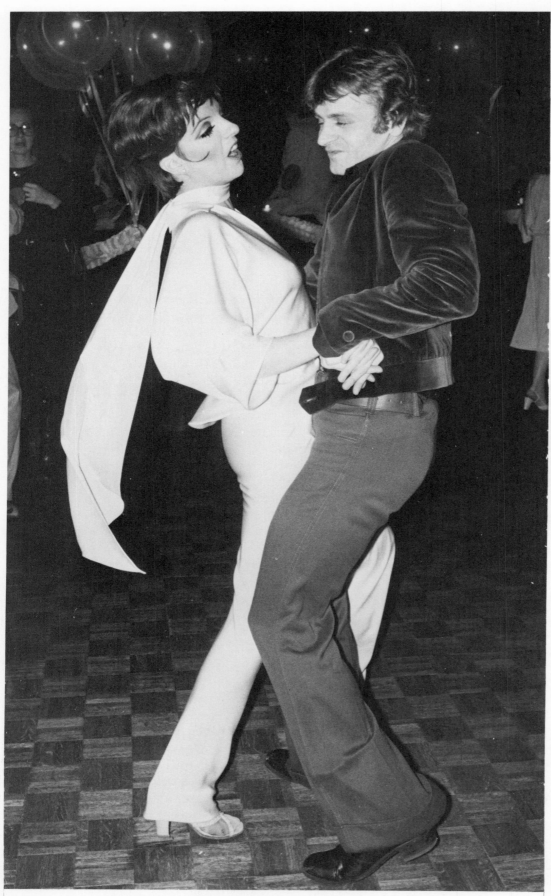

Mikhail Baryshnikov of New York City Ballet does the Hustle with Liza Minnelli.

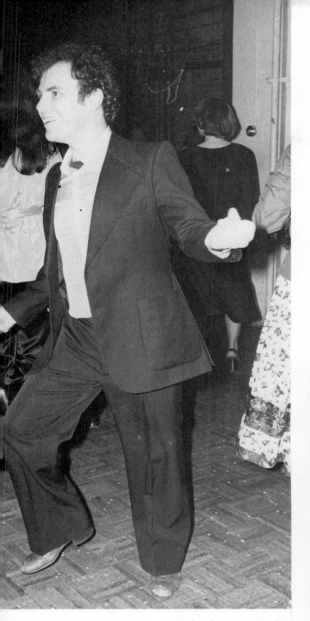

Former Yippie leader Jerry Rubin abandons the barricades for Studio 54.

Mixed disco scene.

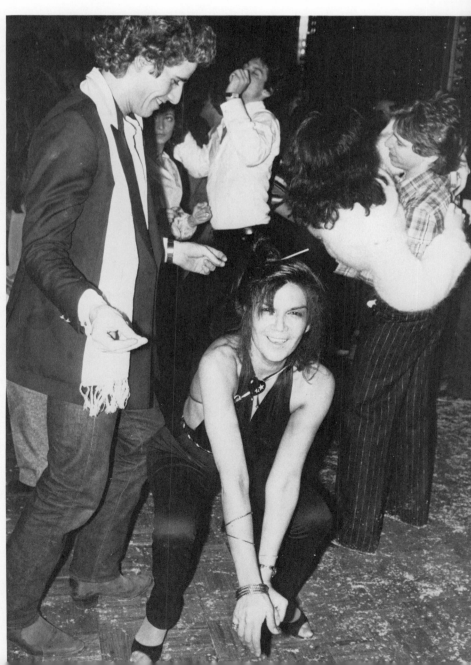

ing to movie screens all across the country. It was confirmation, if any was needed, that dancing together was once again a fact of life on the social scene. The setting was an authentic tough, working class district with an uneasy ethnic mix that had its own edgy glamor and where everybody danced. Of course disco dancing could be seen on television screens any time. The seemingly ageless "American Bandstand" had been duded up in disco glitter and a black equivalent, "Soul Train," had appeared. The couples who, a decade previously, would have been standing apart, were turning and twirling as if the Twist and its ilk had never existed. People were back to a kind of structure in everything.

The teachers in the dance schools and the studios were unabashedly delighted to see the return of touch or smooth dancing which meant a return of dance students to their classroom dance floors. During the sixties they had been as out as the fox trots they taught. A sixties couple doing the Mashed Potatoes might select any of a passel of variations called the Crinkle Cut or the Half Baked or Pan Fried, and who would have dared to challenge anyone doing the Hash Brown? Everything was okay and there was nothing to teach. The dancers made it up as they went along. It may have been riotous fun on the dance floor, but it was a very unhappy time in the studios and school.

The Hustle and Bump meant that there was something to teach again. The dance teachers huffed that smooth dancing had never been away, but might have added that you practically had to look in the haystack to find it. It had never departed from the service academies such as West Point or Annapolis, which prepared their cadets in a traditional way to be accomplished ballroom dancers, as befits proper gentlemen. Smooth dancing had never been abandoned by the older generation who still made regular, weekly pilgrimages to traditional dance halls such as Roseland, in New York, where the familiar rhythms of American and Latin dance bands alternated for the pleasure of those who had never learned to live with the dance anarchy of the sixties. Charity balls and other social functions also never let go of the traditional mix, although the occasional twist might have been thrown into the program. But the impromptu parties of the sixties had far outnumbered any structured events.

The new discos of the seventies bore little resemblance to their sixties counterparts. The early discos had been bizarre enough with their go-go girls and light shows, but they were like Henry Ford's Model T compared to an Indianapolis 500 racer when measured against the newer models of the seventies. Regine's in New York was an extension of a Paris club that cleverly saturated patrons with sound while they danced but kept the level down when they were off the floor. Others invested hundreds of thousands of dollars to create spectacular lighting effects such as a colorful crescent-shaped man in the moon being lowered to sniff from a glittery spoon. The floor itself became a hot checkerboard of lights pulsing in time to the music; fog machines created a sensuous mist for dancers to glow in. The number of discos proliferated as the demand grew steadily.

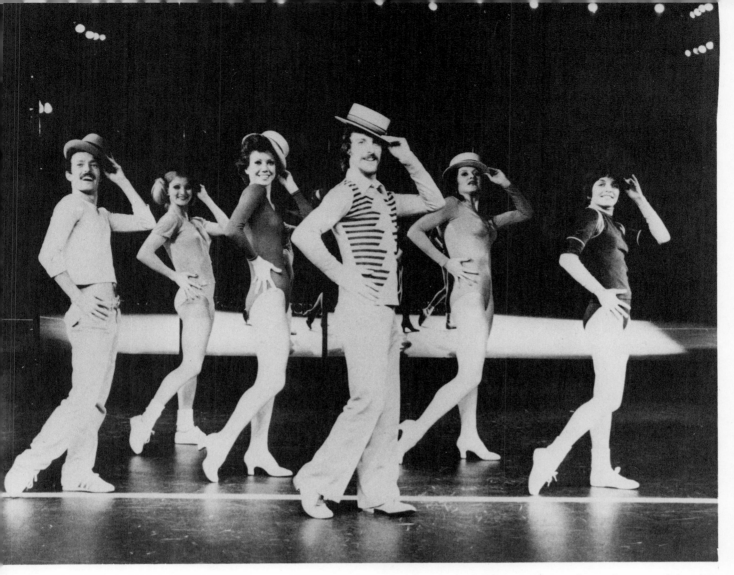

A Chorus Line makes a show out of dancing.

The dance fever became so great that various teachers began to give away free lessons as parts of store promotions. Street fairs provided opportunities to learn the hustle while an enterprising bank had instructors in to teach their depositors on their lunch hours. At the most popular discos, there were nightly disturbances by patrons unable to get in. Topsy-turvy dress codes were followed. In some clubs, men wouldn't be admitted unless in formal dress and in others, the formally dressed would be turned away as they were out of step with the glittery apparel of the regulars. Clubs like Studio 54 selected a crowd on the basis of fame, notoriety, or far out freakiness. People who sprayed their bodies with silver paint rubbed shoulders with those whose pictures appeared in the newspapers or whose names were constantly bandied about by the gossip columnists. The popular life of most of the best discos was short as the incrowd drifted from one hot spot to the next. New places opened up rapidly to replace old ones. They catered to every taste. There were places that specialized in punk rock, where a fight was almost guaranteed. The clientele there dressed in a

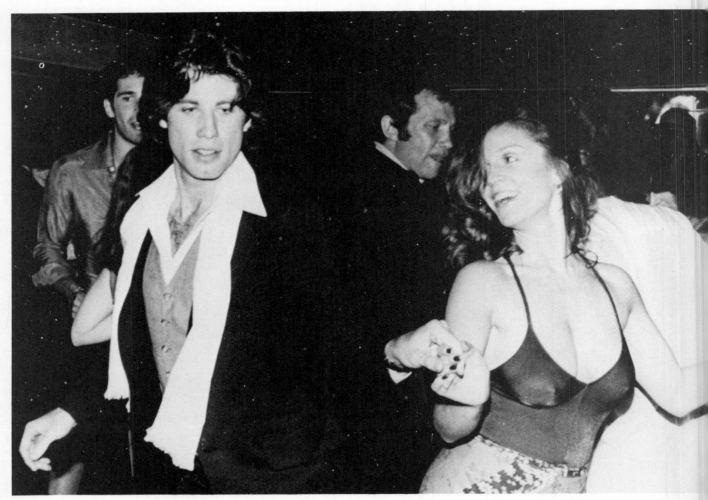

That dancing demon John Travolta takes the floor with Marilu Henner.

tighter, tougher version of the old fifties black leather jacket gangs, and
often pierced their noses or even cheeks and wore safety pins threaded
through the holes. There were gay clubs which maintained restricted
memberships. Dance fever cut across social and sexual lines.

During this time, black dance took an exciting new turn. Thanks to a
dance show, "Soul Train" which aired in 1971, along came a troupe of
dancers called The Lockers who danced the lock-step and all its funky
fantastic variations. The lock required hip-and-knee coordination. The
knee is bent and straightened or "locked" to the beat of the music. The arm
opposite the leg which is locking is thrust forward or upward. Variations
include the Breakdown—a side to side dance—and the Scooby Doo—a
wild high-kicking dance. The dress code here was made up of brightly
striped socks, platform sneakers, and braided, beaded hair in cornrows.
The look was outrageous and funky.

With the new dances were thriving and discos prospered, a quaint little
piece of the past was quietly resurrected. An old custom from pre-World
War I days returned in the form of the *thé dansant,* the tea dance. The

The dance floor that Saturday Night Fever *made famo*

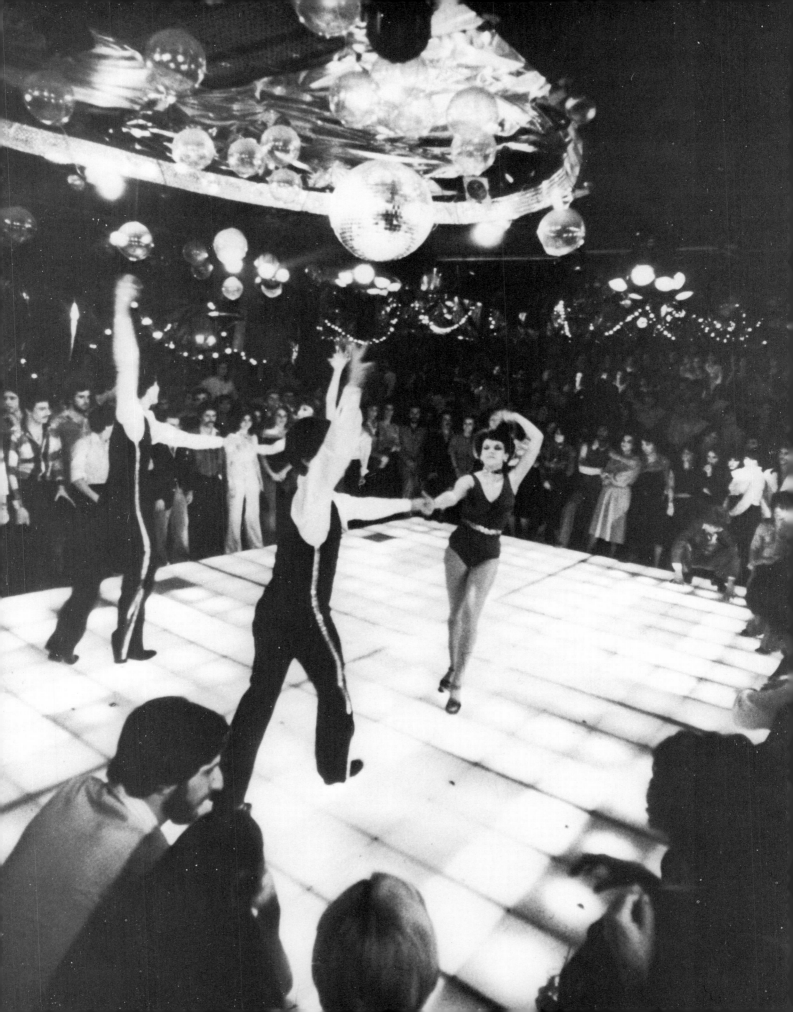

causal visitor to many downtown hotels in cities across the country would find a large inviting sign: "After work take a sentimental journey into the twenties, thirties, and forties with those great big band sounds in our Atrium Park Lobby. Special Tea Dance menu and cash bar. Free admission." In late afternoon, couples glided across the dance floor to live music in hotel lobbies. Other hotels increased the size of their dance floors again to accommodate the smooth dancers and some romantics went right back to the turn of the century for the Viennese waltz.

One such group organized a party of three hundred like-minded devotees, dressed up in white tie and swallow-tailed evening clothes, and invited their ladies to an evening of elegant dancing. Other couples missed the fifties and recreated a prom ambiance by ransacking their closets and dusting off the clothes that they had worn, including those strapless evening gowns that were always a source of hitching anxiety.

Even the marathon dance returned, although in a more benign form at which money was raised for a worthy cause rather than for the surviving couple. The rules were the same but the dancers were considerably younger and their only exposure to the original contest quite possibly had come via the brutal film *They Shoot Horses, Don't They*. The dances they did stemmed from a later period and reflected sixties rock dancing and the Hustle. On Broadway, two musicals, *A Chorus Line* and *Dancin'*, used dance to form the plot and, in general, dance played an increasingly important part in the musical theater.

Schools returned to academic standards that were not based on "relevance" but on excellence, and after the betrayal of Watergate, the government began to open up its own operations for examination. Things were not as settled as they had once seemed but a new integration was beginning to take place. The fifties had seen, in effect, the end of the thirties' philosophy and had also contained the stirrings of the new. Dances of early fifties looked like cooler and less involved versions of traditional social dancing. Men and women still dressed like the ladies and gentlemen of earlier decades but showed a hint of the extreme casualness that flourished in the sixties. Touch dancing was far and away the most common form of dancing.

During the sixties, dance became a solo affair, an expression of the individual. It was free and structureless and too wild for many. Eventually, it became a completely private statement and the dancers hardly moved at all.

The seventies became hesitantly affirmative of older values and attempted to blend them with the newer, liberated attitudes that permeated the sixties. It wasn't a question of turning back the clock and pretending that the sixties hadn't happened but rather of modifying and relaxing the rigid rules of the past that had been logical but had also been applied without much flexibility. Rules were back but it was understood that individuals would want to cut out from time to time.

Dancers of the seventies sought sociability combined with some solo

116

The crowd surges happily.

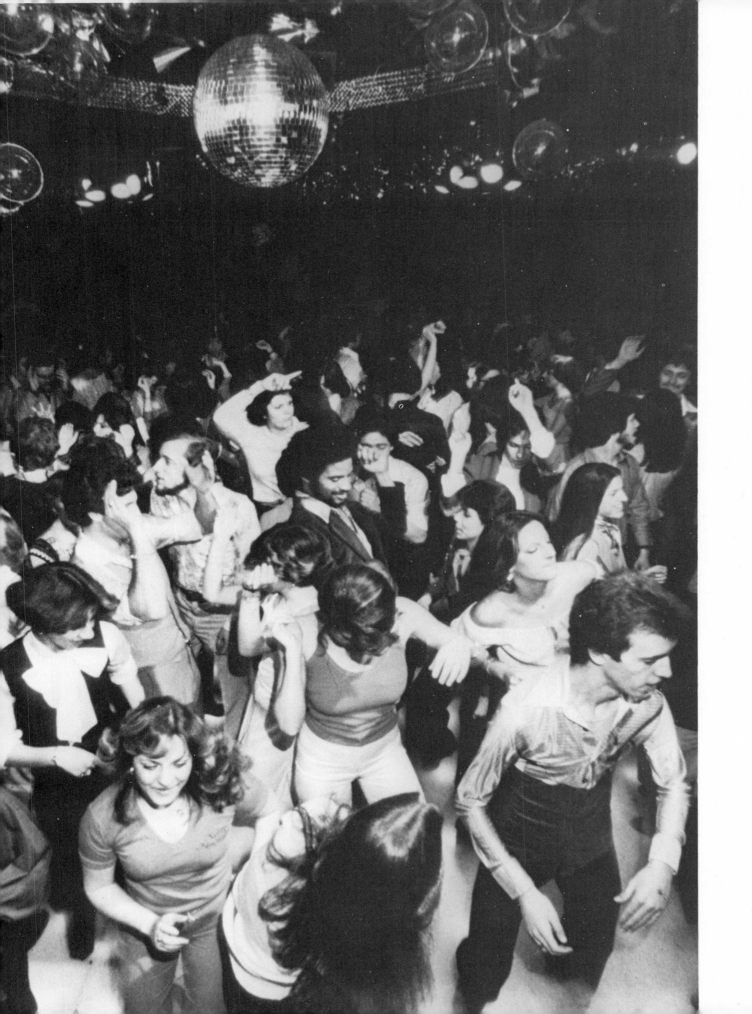

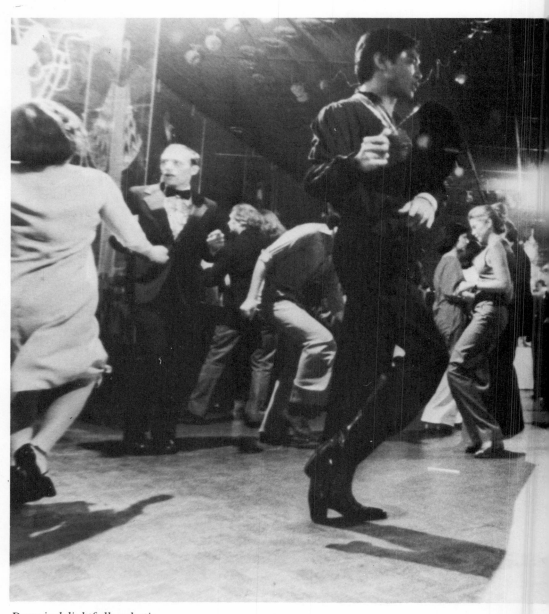

Dress is delightfully eclectic.

maneuverability and they found their answer in the Hustle. It encompassed touch dancing and fancy footwork and combined staying in place with a bit of traveling. The Hustle moved to center stage because it reunited couples on the dance floor while allowing them individuality

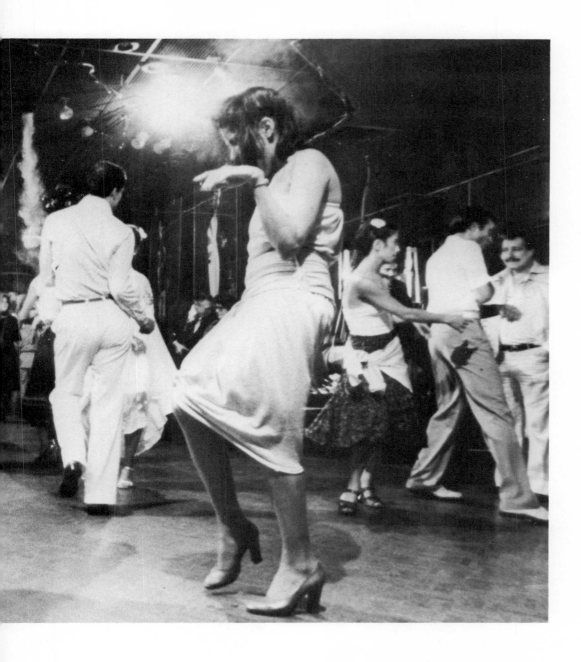

within elastic bounds. Our own Latin dance! The right dance at the right time and it didn't have to be imported. It solved the problem perfectly, and set dance fever in high gear again.

PHOTO CREDITS